Heal
Emotional Eating
For Good

Heal Emotional Eating For Good

Stop comfort eating and start living your dreams

Katrina Love Senn

For more information about Katrina's *Breakthrough Healing Sessions, Yoga and Healing Retreats* and books visit:

www.KatrinaLoveSenn.com

Please note: *Heal Emotional Eating For Good* is not intended to replace medical advice or treatment. If you are dealing with any sort of physical, mental or emotional disorders we suggest that you consult your physician or therapist and use this book under their supervision. Neither the author nor the publisher assumes any responsibility for your improper use of this book.

I dedicate this book to my husband and best friend.

Damien Senn.

Acknowledgements

Thanks to the readers of my first book *Losing Weight is a Healing Journey*. And to those who read, share and comment on my articles.

I love receiving your heart-warming messages of transformation and healing. Thanks for sharing your experiences, wisdom and insight.

I am grateful for my healing clients and yoga students. Witnessing your courage to stretch and grow has inspired this book.

I would also like to acknowledge and thank my family. Especially my Mum and Dad, Sandra and Peter. And my Mother and Father-in-law, Pauline and Gary. Your love, encouragement and support mean the world to me.

I also want to extend gratitude to the many libraries, cafés and countries this book was written in.

This book contains the inspiration of Australia, Cyprus, Greece, Indonesia, Italy, New Zealand, Spain, Thailand, United Kingdom and the United States of America weaved into its pages.

Finally, I would like to give special acknowledgement to Damien Senn, my husband, partner and soul mate.

Thank you for being by my side for every step of this book creation journey.

Love Katrina xo

Contents

Introduction

"The day came when the risk to remain tight in a bud was more painful than the risk it took to blossom."

~ Anaïs Nin

For many women, the idea of being able to *Heal Emotional Eating For Good* is an impossible notion.

It is hard enough dealing with life's external demands. Let alone address the terrain of our innermost thoughts and feelings. Right?

The dieting industry will have you believe that emotional eating is a problem to be fought and struggled against.

It is this very struggle that perpetuates an unnecessary cycle of guilt, shame and suffering so many women privately endure.

Now I want to assure you that struggle does have its place on any true journey of transformation. In fact, I spent nearly a decade struggling with emotional eating myself.

What I'm about to share with you in this book is another way.

Emotional eating is not something that you need to fight against like you have been led to believe. This ongoing battle only serves to tighten the knot.

The possibility I want to share with you is that you can *Heal Emotional Eating For Good.* You can do this by using simple yet powerful healing tools just as I have done.

This book has been written for the woman who is tired of the struggle. And is finally ready and willing to move beyond it...

Am I talking to the right lady here?

Okay great. Then please keep reading...

So why did I write this book?

Heal Emotional Eating For Good is my second book.

I decided to write this book to continue the conversation I started in my first book.

In **Losing Weight is a Healing Journey**, I shared how I lost over 60 pounds naturally without diets, drugs or deprivation (in case you're wondering, that's around 25 kilograms or 50 tubs of butter!).

I also managed to heal chronic health conditions I had suffered with since childhood. These included asthma and eczema.

It was a deep and at times humbling process for me to open up and share intimate details of my journey in my first book. I felt encouraged and inspired by all the lovely feedback I received.

Many women bought the book because they wanted to heal their relationship with food. As well as themselves.

I have a first hand knowledge of this desire to heal. A few days before my 20th birthday, my body completely broke down.

When I hit rock bottom, it became clear to me that healing was the only path that made any sense.

I couldn't see any point in trying to implement yet another 'Band-Aid' solution.

What I was looking for was something that could free me from my mental and emotional prison.

I also wanted to finally feel at home within my body.

If you are reading this book, it is very possible you may have hit a similar breaking point yourself?

By being willing to go on my healing journey I was able to restore my health. I also freed myself from the need to use food as a constant source of comfort and protection.

So what does this book offer?

Heal Emotional Eating For Good offers you a simple, yet effective set of healing tools. You can use these tools to heal your emotional eating. You can also free yourself from the guilt, shame and loss of self-confidence that comes with it.

In this book I will be sharing how you can use emotional eating as a pathway to self-discovery and healing.

I will reveal how you can nourish and nurture your physical body. You can do this whilst letting go of the thoughts and feelings that no longer serve you. I will also reveal how you can build an honest and loving relationship with yourself.

This book will help you to release the struggle of emotional eating for good. It will help you to love more, to soften and to heal.

The gentle healing tools I offer in this book are ones that anyone can utilise. You can use them to access previously unobtainable breakthroughs. This can happen even if you have been an emotional eater your entire life.

Of course you don't need to apply all the healing tools at once. Just pick and choose the ones that feel timely and relevant for you.

What this book *'isn't'* about.

This book *isn't* about changing your life overnight. Nor is it about gaining exclusive access to some 'pill-shaped miracle cure'. The best breakthroughs come from committing to a process of self-exploration and transformation.

One thing I want to make clear is that this book is not about handing your authority over to anyone else. If you are waiting for someone to 'wave a magic wand' and solve all your problems, then this *isn't* the right book for you.

If you are ready to release the stress that causes emotional eating, then please keep reading. This book contains many treasures for you to discover…

The real answers are inside of you.

This book doesn't proclaim to contain all the answers on emotional eating. The reason it doesn't is because I do not have all the answers. The most important distinctions you will make on this journey aren't the ones others give you. They are the ones you make for yourself.

You do not need to have a clinical understanding of emotional eating to heal. I didn't and still managed to do so.

The healing journey is all about learning how to trust and follow your inner teacher. Also known as your 'in-tuition'.

It's about turning down the volume of the voices on the 'outside' so you can hear your true voice on the 'inside'.

As you develop your intuition, your ability to create meaningful change will flourish.

The answers you are looking for are inside of you. My intention with this book is to inspire and guide you to find them.

Getting the most out of this book.

This book has been designed to be a gateway of self-discovery. It's more guidebook than instruction manual. To get the most out of it I encourage you to stay open, curious and playful with the material.

You wouldn't be reading this book unless a deeper part of you already knew it could work for you.

There are no 'shoulds' or 'musts' on this journey. There is no pressure and no expectations. The beauty about this is that you get to decide what you take from it and how far you will take things as well.

Always remember that this is your healing process. You can take it at your own pace and work with it in a way that feels natural and comfortable for you.

Working from this place of ease and grace is the key that opens the door to healing.

An invitation to heal.

Heal Emotional Eating For Good is a personal invitation to start your healing journey.

In this book I will be revealing how you can use your emotional eating as a tool for healing. Many of the distinctions I share have come from healing my emotional eating patterns.

The book also benefits from the many *Breakthrough Healing Sessions* I have conducted over the years. And the *Yoga and Healing Retreats* I have run throughout the world.

In this book I will be sharing inspirational stories from women just like you. I will also be sharing some of my personal stories as well.

From 'emotional eating' to 'emotional freedom'.

Emotional eating provides a fascinating lens to explore your life through. I believe it is something that should be celebrated rather than shrouded in shame.

Your life is always inviting you to step into a greater expression of who you are. Emotional eating is your unique guidance system that will help show you the way.

The healing journey always finds you at the perfect time. This path is not one you can force upon the unwilling. It has to be something you feel called to explore through your own experience.

The healing journey was one I was compelled to walk for myself. It wasn't always easy but it was most definitely worthwhile.

And now it is my deepest honour to share what I have learnt with you.

If you have weight concerns, I recommend you also read my first book *Losing Weight is a Healing Journey.*

It makes an excellent companion to the material I will be sharing with you in this book.

You can Heal Emotional Eating For Good.

When I was sick, tired and overweight, it was almost impossible for me to imagine losing all my excess weight. Or heal my emotional eating for that matter.

It was even harder to imagine I would one day write a book sharing what I discovered on my healing journey.

And writing a second book... Well, that was beyond my wildest imagination.

One thing I have learnt from going on this journey is our challenges become the doorway to our dreams.

I healed my emotional eating for good. And I know if you are curious and willing that you can too.

My hope is this book will help you to access the courage necessary to address what *isn't* working in your life.

I also hope it gives you the confidence to acknowledge and expand what *is*.

Allow this book to become a trusted friend. Turn to it whenever you are looking for insight and inspiration.

Of all the many millions of books written across time, this book has found its way to you.

I want to assure you it has come into your experience for a very good reason.

And that reason will become clear as you turn these pages...

Chapter One – My Story of Emotional Eating

"Blessed are the hearts that can bend; they shall never be broken."

~ Albert Camus

My path to breakdown

"Healing happens when the untold stories of our darkest nights are set free into the light of day."

~ Katrina Love Senn

It was the night I will never forget.

I was studying in a coastal town in New Zealand. My second year of university was days away from commencing.

I had spent my first year at university living in one of the 'off campus' student dormitories.

Our college had a proud tradition of helping first year students transition into university life.

There were around 100 students, both male and female, who lived there. We were each given our own room, three meals a day and a quiet place to study.

After our first year, we were expected to find our own independent accommodation. This was so we could create space for the next intake of 'freshers'.

College life reminded me of living at boarding school. Although it granted me a lot more freedom, I longed for the independence of living in my own flat share.

I started the process of looking for a new place to live with a group of university friends.

We trawled the colourful array of student accommodation the area had to offer.

Finally we submitted an application on a three-storey town house. It was newly constructed and situated in a quiet cul-de-sac.

Much to our delight, we soon found out we had been successful.

A cause for celebration.

It was our first Saturday in our new house and there was a buzz of excitement in the air.

Students from all over the country descended upon the town after the summer break.

We decided our new house was a cause for celebration. So we invited some friends around for an impromptu house warming.

Everyone was feeling merry and in the mood for a good time.

When nightfall came someone suggested we move the party to a nearby student pub.

As people headed for the door, I realised I had left my jacket upstairs.

So I told them I would grab it and catch them up.

I then climbed the two flights of stairs to my room.

I was a little tipsier than I had first thought.

Rather than grab my jacket, I decided I needed a quick lay-down first.

I must have fallen straight to sleep.

My next memory was hearing my bedroom light being switched off and my door being pushed shut.

I opened my eyes and there lurking in the shadows was a male silhouette.

As my sight adjusted I could see it was Jake. [1]

---

[1] The names in this story have been changed.

Something was not right.

A wave of panic crushed over me.

I had met Jake for the first time earlier at the party.   He was the boyfriend of a girl at university called Brenda.

Apart from playing rugby and working on a sheep farm, I knew little about him.

Jake broke the ice with a slew of incoherent slurs. My mind sobered instantly.

Beads of sweat formed at the base of my spine and my heart thumped with distress.

I wanted to run but a paralysis took over me.

Trapped in my room, there was no way I could escape.

With his misguided pleasantries out of the way, Jake unbuttoned his shirt.

He then scrambled his way onto the bed like he was entering a rugby scrum.

The stench of liquor emanating from his pores filled my nostrils with revulsion.

Once he had found his position, he lunged forward and began trying to win me over me.

As I struggled against Jake's unwanted advances, my defiance was met with an overpowering force.

He smothered me with his size as his coarse hands grabbed at my body.

As he affirmed his stronghold, his gaze fixated upon me.

It was like he was almost daring me to try and contest his physical prowess.

I had never felt so scared in my entire life.

It was as if my body had been taken hostage by fear itself.

In a desperate attempt to halt his drunken antics I spluttered…

"Brenda loves you Jake and I know you love her too. Let's go and find the others down at the pub."

I cringed as the words tumbled out of my mouth.

Given the unfolding circumstances, it was a ludicrous line.

A smirk lit up Jake's face.

I turned desperate.

Instinctively I knew I had to keep talking.

I couldn't think of anything else to say so I repeated the words,

"Brenda loves you Jake and I know you love her too."

Jake again dismissed my plea and intensified his advances.

With all the might I had left within me I cried out one last time,

"Brenda loves you Jake…"

And then as if by magic, something popped and his encroachment ceased.

He sat upright on the side of the bed facing the wall.

It was over…

I took a moment to catch my breath.

I wiped the tears from my eyes and walked over to the other side of the room.

I was thankful to have escaped the incident unharmed.

I straightened my clothes. I then put my jacket on as if it were the protective shield I needed to keep me safe.

I looked over at Jake. He was crouched over, holding his head up with his hands. With my arms folded, I requested one last time that we go find the others at the pub.

He put his shirt back on and with very little resistance I walked him down the stairs and across the road.

A couple of friends noticed my late arrival and asked what had taken me so long. I was in a total state of shock and pretended as if nothing had happened.

I never saw Jake again.

I figured he must have returned home after a weekend of partying. And carried on with his life on the farm.

***

I woke up the next day feeling tender.

I confided with a friend about what had happened.

I felt awkward and embarrassed about the incident.

The last thing I wanted was for anyone else to find out about it. So I asked her to keep it a secret.

After hearing what I had to say, she concluded I had two choices:

Choice 1: Tell Brenda about the whole episode.
Choice 2: Pretend as if nothing had happened.

I must admit I was surprised to hear her say I had 'choices'.

To me it seemed like I had no choice at all.

The last thing I wanted to do was dramatise the incident further.

Chatting with Brenda would only add to the distress I already felt inside.

And besides, would she even believe me?

Or worse still, would she somehow blame me by saying I had encouraged the whole thing?

After all, it would be my word against his.

By the end of our chat, I'd convinced myself I was fine.

All I wanted to do was forget about what had happened so I could get on with my life.

As I lay in my bed later that night, I kept going over the events of the previous night in my mind.

I couldn't contain the overwhelming feelings brewing up inside of me.

I felt so stupid and ashamed.

I mean how could I have been so foolish and naïve?

I was angry I had let myself get into that kind of situation.

Rather than vent my anger outwards, I turned it inwards.

I criticised myself in the darkness with my own harsh and unforgiving thoughts.

This desperate self-attack continued long into the night until I was exhausted.

I vowed to bury the incident in the recesses of my being and never speak of it again.

I then drifted off to sleep…

Emotional eating and the sensitive woman.

Like many emotional eaters, I was a sensitive and empathic child. I possessed the ability to feel pain deeply, both my own as well as others.

Due to these sensitivities I took most things personally. This tendency had a detrimental impact upon my self-esteem and self-worth.

My parents did an amazing job taking care of the practical needs of my 'outer world'. What I found challenging was navigating the thoughts and feelings of my 'inner world'.

As a teenager I felt like I was different to everyone else and found it tricky fitting in. I had always suspected that there must be something wrong with me, yet I wasn't quite sure what that something was.

I never felt as if I was 'good enough' at anything. Even well meaning feedback felt like criticism. I wasn't at the top of my class, despite being quite studious and I felt out of place on the sporting field.

The weight that had crept its way onto my body insulated me from a seemingly cruel and insensitive world. This fleshy barrier became the perfect place to hide my feelings of inadequacy and shame.

I did my best to compensate for my perceived shortcomings by being a 'good girl'. I helped others wherever I could and became a natural 'people pleaser'.

I attended to the needs of others whilst neglecting my own. I avoided conflict by trying to keep everybody around me happy.

The one place I did feel at home was in the kitchen. I had a passion for cooking and loved to delight family and friends with birthday cakes and other treats. My baking skills gained me the love, attention and approval I longed for.

I found a real comfort in food. Emotional eating became my way of dealing with things that overwhelmed me.

This pattern started out innocently. By the time I commenced university it was a well-honed coping strategy.

My emotional eating went into over-drive.

When university recommenced I carried on with my life.

My family had a well-oiled pattern of avoiding conflict. Growing up I had often heard comments like 'don't rock the boat', 'don't make a fuss out of nothing' and 'grin and bear it'.

Repressing my feelings had become something I saw no reason to question as a young adult.

Rather than deal with the Jake thing, I avoided it. I also avoided anything else that could trigger awkward and uncomfortable feelings. This included parties, alcohol and boys.

My eating patterns became erratic. I had stopped cooking at home and ate most of my meals on the go. Any time I felt difficult emotions flaring up, I would use food to stuff them back down.

Food had always brought such pleasure to me growing up. Somehow it had morphed into something very private and shameful.

The sweetness I used to experience in my life had all but disappeared from my daily existence. Instead I self-medicated my pain with coffee, chocolate and sugar coated treats.

Of course, it didn't matter how much I ate, none of it could fill the emotional void that was consuming me from the inside.

I began to experience episodes of anxiety and depression.

My soul was crying out for support and guidance. I was still in a state of denial about what had happened. I felt vulnerable with no safe place to turn.

Each morning before heading to class, I would put on loose clothing to hide my body and a happy face to mask my pain.

I would then dash to my lectures, tutorials and other engagements.

In hindsight, all I was doing was running from myself.

And then one day my body broke down.

It was days before my 20th birthday when my body broke down. The traumatic experience with Jake, combined with my stressful university schedule had exhausted my nervous system.

I finally 'hit the wall' whilst attending a student conference in Australia. I had travelled there to deliver a speech to a room full of my peers. I was terrified of public speaking and 'being seen'. I'd spent weeks anticipating my speech and my body was feeling the strain.

On the morning after my talk, I woke up unable to move my body. It felt like my glands were breathing fire. My eyelids were swollen shut and hundreds of mini cold sores had appeared on my face overnight.

I was a complete mess. My 'emotional well' had run dry and my physical reserves were depleted. I felt empty inside with nothing more to give.

Making the choice to heal.

I returned home to New Zealand and spent the next couple of months bedridden and sleeping for up to 18 hours per day.

I underwent a series of routine medical tests. The results showed I was sick and my body was out of balance. What was less clear was what I was going to do about it.

My doctor explained she wanted to treat my symptoms with experimental medication.

I intuitively felt this wasn't the right course of action for me.

The prescription I needed was to rest, nourish and re-balance my body.

I wanted to re-connect with the acceptance, forgiveness and peace that lived inside of me.

My days of using emotional eating as a coping strategy had ended.

And my healing journey had only just begun…

The 3 phases of the healing journey

"My advice to you is not to undertake the spiritual path. It is too difficult, too long, and is too demanding. I suggest you ask for your money back, and go home. This is not a picnic. It is really going to ask everything of you. So, it is best not to begin. However, if you do begin, it is best to finish."

~ Chögyam Trungpa

Emotional eating always happens for a reason. When you know what to look for, this reason will reveal itself to you.

Before diving further into this book, let's take a moment to explore the remaining structure of it.

There are three distinct phases on the journey to *Heal Emotional Eating For Good*. These are…

Phase 1: Emotional Eating
Phase 2: Emotional Healing
Phase 3: Emotional Freedom

These are the same three phases I had to navigate on my healing journey.

I have used the lotus flower to symbolise these three phases (see diagram on the following page).

The lotus flower to me is a symbol of the growth and transformation that is possible through healing.

The lotus flower begins its first phase of life in the mud at the bottom of the pond as it takes root.

In its second phase, the stem begins to grow through the murky water and its green leaves start to form.

In the final phase, the lotus blossom emerges out of the water revealing its full glory.

With greater awareness you too will be able to *Heal Emotional Eating For Good*.

And like the beautiful lotus, when you keep moving towards the light, you will blossom into all you can be.

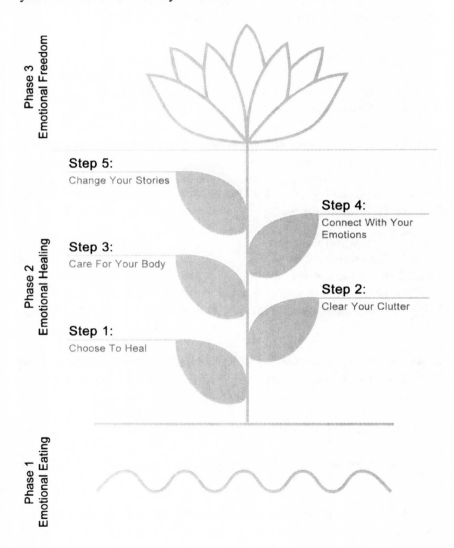

Phase 1: Emotional Eating.

Symbol: The lotus root.

Phase 1 is where the majority of women find themselves on the healing journey.

This phase is an unconscious one and because of this it can also be very challenging to break out of.

I was stuck in this phase for most of my teenage life.

This phase can initially be quite joyous and carefree.

The expression 'blissfully unaware' is a great way to describe this state.

In this phase, there is little awareness of the thoughts and feelings at the root of emotional eating.

There is also a lack of awareness of the many different healing tools available as well.

A woman in this phase is vulnerable to the sophisticated marketing tactics used by supermarkets. And fast food chains.

These corporations profit from keeping women trapped in this unconscious phase of development.

Emotional eating is a sign she does not yet have all the answers. It is a call to awaken her intuition and step into her true power.

A woman is quite within her rights to stay here if she chooses.

However the downstream consequences that arise out of emotional eating are inescapable.

If it continues without exploration, it can become more confusing, frustrating and painful.

To start healing emotional eating for good, it is necessary to look within and make the choice to heal.

Phase 2: Emotional Healing.

Symbol: The lotus leaf.

Phase 2 is a big growth phase. It is here where a woman will start to look for deeper answers about her emotional eating.

This phase begins when a woman makes the 'choice to heal'. To do this it is essential she commits to doing something different.

Phase 1 begins in bliss and becomes more painful. Phase 2 begins in some kind of pain and becomes more blissful.

Women in this phase may still use emotional eating to deal with stress. When they do, it is with an active awareness that brings growth, self-knowledge and healing.

This phase of self-enquiry can often be initiated through deep frustration or pain. My self-enquiry began when my body moved so far out of balance that it broke down.

For other women this phase may start with a career crisis, a relationship breakdown or even the loss of a loved one. It can also emerge out of being 'fed up' of living life on other people's terms. Or even from a desire to live a more fun, authentic and expressive life.

A woman in this phase takes responsibility for her thoughts, feelings and actions. She will start to connect with her inner power and have the courage to question social norms.

She will seek out and experiment with healing tools to release stress and heal past hurts. She will also invest in the support, guidance and mentorship she needs.

This phase of the healing journey is non-linear. Sometimes women can experience spontaneous healings that free them from emotional eating.

For others, it can take a longer period of exploration and integration.

This phase ends when a woman no longer needs emotional eating to cope with the stress of her everyday life.

Phase 3: Emotional Freedom.

Symbol: The lotus blossom.

Phase 3 is the bonus stage of the emotional healing journey.

It begins and ends in bliss. In this phase a woman reveals her true self and shines.

A woman in phase 3 treats herself with a deep love, honour and respect.

She will have cultivated a healthy and balanced lifestyle that is an authentic expression of her values.

She enjoys the sacred bond that exists between her mind and body. She has learnt to 'feel her feelings' rather than 'feed them'.

She is self-aware and knows how to get her soul needs met in a healthy and life affirming way.

A woman in this phase of development has healed the root causes of her emotional eating. She has become immune to the tricks used by food marketers.

She has worked out how to say 'yes' to the things that bring her joy. And 'no' to the things that bring her unnecessary stress and anxiety.

She views food as a source of nourishment and pleasure. She can enjoy it without guilt, self-punishment or excessive control.

A woman in this phase feels at home in her body.

She has come to know and cherish her feminine power and encourages other women to do the same.

She is an inspiration to all those around her. She is attuned to the precious miracle of life and commits to living fully.

She radiates beauty and confidence from the inside out and has become a beacon of light for the world.

PHASE 1:

Emotional Eating

Chapter Two – The Outer World of Emotional Eating

"People are fed by the food industry, which pays no attention to health, and are treated by the health industry, which pays no attention to food."

~ Wendell Berry

The world we live in

"In our fast-forward culture, we have lost the art of eating well. Food is often little more than fuel to pour down the hatch while doing other stuff."

~ Carl Honoré

I graduated from university with an honours degree in Marketing.

The reward for my toil was a fancy cap and gown. I was also given a paper scroll with my name on it and a sizable student debt accruing interest daily.

Motivated to free myself from the ominous financial legacy of my degree, I began my job search in earnest.

My two great passions were travel and food. I hoped my first real job would relate to either one of these areas.

My search of the graduate job market yielded two potential opportunities.

The first position was working for one of the world's top airlines. The second was in a food division of a leading multi-national.

Both jobs were well paid. They also had great prospects for career advancement and travel. I knew both positions would meet with the approval of my family and friends.

My personal preference was to work for the airline. It seemed much more glamourous and exciting.

I sent in my application and made my way through to the last round of interviews at the airline.

A few days after the interview, I received a rejection letter.

It appeared as if life had made the decision for me, so I took the job at the multi-national.

My first day on the job.

My graduate placement was in an area sales role within the company's ice cream division.

Having spent the previous few years healing my emotional eating, the irony of the job was not wasted on me.

When I took the position, I thought there might be scope for me to share my healing story. I was also keen to inspire the introduction of healthier food options.

The folly of my innocence was soon revealed. On my job induction I discovered the focus of my role was to help the company to sell more processed ice cream.

It dawned on me I had made a huge mistake.

Mindful of my financial obligations, I committed to doing my best and to learn as much as I could.

I was assigned to a sales territory and given a brand new company car.

I did my best to enjoy this rare graduate perk, but for some reason the 'new car smell' left me feeling queasy.

My customers were independent corner stores and petrol stations. I also serviced a few large supermarkets as well.

I had three main strategies to increase sales. These were improving signage, maximising retail space and keeping the freezers clean and well stocked.

I spent most of my time on the road.

I would also call into the office to write up customer sales reports and catch up on administration.

The sales office contained a large freezer filled with all the latest ice cream samples.

On the job challenges.

My job selling processed ice cream held many challenges.

Firstly, I had made the choice to stop eating 'fake foods' while I was healing my body[2]. I found it uncomfortable to have to decline invitations from my co-workers to try the latest ice creams.

Secondly, visiting convenience stores was confronting for me. To heal my body, I decided to limit my exposure to supermarkets. This was so I could avoid their marketing tricks. I instead favoured local farmers markets, green grocers and health food stores.

Thirdly, I was the only woman on our sales team. Most of our informal team building exercises involved alcohol. Needless to say, I was teased and mocked for being 'a girl'.

The most challenging thing about my role was selling something I didn't believe in. To keep my job, I had to promote processed ice creams to my customers, even though I no longer ate them myself.

Now rest assured I am someone who believes in the virtues of ice cream. I just prefer ice cream made from natural ingredients.

Despite the challenges, the one thing that made my job worthwhile was my manager. He had a gift for encouraging and developing his team.

After my first nine months on the job, he announced he had been head hunted by another company. He said his replacement would be responsible for implementing the latest company research.

At his farewell, he thanked us all for our service and wished us well for the future.

---

[2] In *Losing Weight is a Healing Journey* I define 'fake foods' as food that has been heavily processed and removed from its natural state.

Customers for life.

The head office marketing team presented their strategic plan.   It detailed how our division could increase profits.

One of their main recommendations was to move beyond the concept of 'repeat customers'.   What they wanted to do instead was create 'customers for life'.

To achieve this, they said the company would focus upon forging strong bonds with children.

They envisioned our products becoming an indistinguishable part of a child's world.

They said we would partner with toy manufacturers, publishers, merchandisers, television producers and product placement experts.

My new manager described the marketing plan as *"ingenious"*.   He then shared his eager anticipation and excitement for the roll out.

Of course there was no mention of the downstream costs to society for rolling out this strategy.

I was appalled.

In that moment, I knew my days selling ice cream were over.

I didn't care how much student debt I still had.   I didn't want to be part of a business that shaped children into being life long consumers.

I knew exactly how hard it had been for me to break free of my own food related compulsions.

I couldn't bear the thought of playing a role in handing out similar fates to innocent children.

It became clear to me that I was not born to perpetuate the problem.

I was here to be a part of the solution...

Become aware of the invisible structures

"Until you make the unconscious conscious, it will direct your life and you will call it fate."

~ *C. G. Jung*

Despite what I felt at the time, my days selling ice cream was not some kind of horrible mistake.

I came to see the experience as an incredible gift. It gave me the opportunity to pull back the curtain. I saw the secret world that works against the health aspirations of women like you and me.

I was able to see how my emotional eating challenges weren't my fault as I had been led to believe.

I wasn't an emotional eater because I was a weak person or lacked willpower. The full picture was much bigger than this.

What I could now see was that I was up against a sophisticated multi-billion dollar industry. An industry focused upon getting unsuspecting consumers hooked on fake foods. And this table had been tilted against me since birth.

This is a world where clever marketers plotted their latest profit seeking manoeuvres. These initiatives were waged against members of society most vulnerable to their ploys.

The game is to get consumers dependent upon their fake food products. This is so their shareholders can feed on the profits.

They achieve this by using techniques so pervasive that they are difficult for the unaware mind to detect.

My experience helped me not to take these games personally. These companies weren't targeting 'me' specifically.

They were targeting people 'like me'. People not yet wise enough to see through their fancy promotional gimmicks.

Addiction and the profit seeking motive.

Could you imagine trying to solve a drug problem at a user level? Whilst turning a 'blind eye' to the actions and motives of the dealers.

It wouldn't be much of a solution right?

Drug cartel profits rely upon techniques to lure people to try their products. They do this with the intent to create addicts. This often occurs at an age before their clientele are able to make informed decisions.

In a similar way, corporate profits rely upon strategies to get consumers 'hooked' on fake food.

And why? Well the simple answer is that it makes financial sense for them to do so.

My work colleagues were regular everyday guys 'doing their jobs'. They were good people. They all had dreams of paying off their student loans and mortgages. And they wanted to create a better future for themselves and their families.

The trouble with the multinational I worked for was that it had no innate sense of moral or social responsibility.

They prioritised their profits over creating a healthy society for everyone to enjoy and be proud of.

It was a big realisation.

It helped me to drop into an even deeper level of compassion and self-forgiveness for my own struggle.

I had been up against a formidable foe. My innocence and naiveté had been my downfall.

The truth is I didn't stand a chance.

And neither, I am assuming, did you...

How did we get here?

"You may encounter many defeats, but you must not be defeated. In fact, it may be necessary to encounter the defeats, so you can know who you are, what you can rise from, how you can still come out of it."

~ Maya Angelou

Charles Dickens, in his classic novel 'A Tale of Two Cities' wrote *"It was the best of times, it was the worst of times…"*

Was Dickens looking through a crystal ball and describing the world we find ourselves in? He could well have been.

The world of today is an incredible juxtaposition.

Women have never had access to so many tools for transformation and healing. Nor have there been so many temptations and distractions to lead us astray.

It's nice to imagine we could all somehow escape the 'ills of human progress' and return to a simpler time.

The reality for each of us is that our soul mission is to be here on earth now. Navigating both the trials and blessings of the modern world.

One of the biggest challenges of our time is emotional eating. As we are about to discover, the epidemic we witness today is a recent phenomenon in the human experience.

There are three key 'outer world' conditions that contribute to the incidence of emotional eating.

These are:

1. Industrialisation of food production.
2. Mass urbanisation.
3. A culture of overconsumption.

1. Industrialisation of food production.

If you were a pre-industrial woman, there would have been many things inhibiting your emotional eating.

Chronic hunger, widespread malnutrition and even periodic famines were the norm. This was true for most of the world's population up until the late 19th century.[3]

Food scarcity meant that it would be difficult for emotional eating to turn chronic.

As a woman, you would have been the primary caregiver and nurturer of the family.

In times of food scarcity, it is likely you would have put the nutritional needs of others above your own. Including those of your children, husband and parents.

Chances are you would have been involved in the food cultivation process as most women were. The food you ate would have also been from natural and organic production methods.

Contrast this with the world we find ourselves in today. Never before has there been such an abundance of food on planet earth.

To maximise yields, we have moved away from local and organic farming methods.

Food producers today focus upon large-scale industrial production, manufacturing and distribution.

---

[3] Many people in the world are still chronically undernourished. The UN 2012 publication 'The State of Food Insecurity in the World 2012' reports that 870 million people are undernourished. Of these, 854 million people live in developing countries. And 16 million people live in developed countries.

Much of the world's food is grown on monoculture farms. They are designed to increase efficiency and optimise bottom lines.

This often comes at the expense of consumer health and the environment.

Many fields are sown using genetically modified seeds engineered not to reproduce. This practice decreases biodiversity whilst increasing crop susceptibility to pests and disease.

To counteract these problems, pesticides, herbicides and fungicides are used. These chemicals destroy soil fertility, pollute water supplies and poison our food.

Artificial preservatives, colours, flavours and additives are used in the food manufacturing process. This cuts costs and increases shelf life.

Adding these toxic substances into our food chain have increased health concerns. It has also contributed to epidemic levels of emotional eating and obesity.

The techniques used to farm livestock are also alarming. Mass farmed animals live their short lives trapped in cages.

They are often injected with hormones to increase their growth speeds. And given antibiotics to counteract poor living conditions.

Our global food distribution system creates extreme levels of wastage and food miles.

Most food packaging is non-biodegradable and ends up in landfills, rivers and oceans.

Although this all seems pretty heavy, there are grass roots movements working to educate consumers.

Many are reversing the ills of an industrialised food production system.

More people are becoming aware of the benefits of choosing local and organic food. There has also been a resurgence of people growing their own food and herbs.

2. Mass urbanisation.

We have seen huge population migrations around the world over the past hundred years. People have been moving away from rural areas into high-density urban dwellings.

For most women it is no longer necessary to toil in the fields, tend to livestock or forage to survive. In fact, due to mass urbanisation, it's no longer even possible.

One of the unfortunate consequences of urbanisation is emotional eating. People have been turning to fake foods to cope with the stress of their lives.

The World Health Organisation estimated that 54% of the global population lived in urban environments in 2014. This figure is up from 34% in 1960 and continues to grow.

The global population has also exploded. In 1900 the world's population was approximately 1.5 billion people. In 2015, the population stood closer to 7.2 billion.

Urbanisation has facilitated great advances in wealth creation. It has also expanded living standards for many. This has occurred by moving workers out of agriculture and into the service economy.

It is also worth noting that urbanisation has come with challenges.

Some of the bigger issues related to urbanisation include: overcrowding, unsustainable development, traffic congestion, pollution, environmental degradation, natural resource misuse and decreasing levels of public health.

Some of the key issues for the emotional eater include more sedentary lifestyles, longer working hours, job insecurity, longer commutes, financial pressure, changes in eating habits, escalating health costs and the increased availability of fake food.

These issues have all contributed to the stress women experience today. This in turn has led to alarming levels of emotional eating and also obesity.

3. A culture of overconsumption.

The food industry today is 'big business'. And the guiding philosophy of big business is to maximise profits.

Industrialised food production in the West means we no longer worry about the 'under supply' of food. Today it is the 'over supply' of food that is creating serious implications.

Food has never been so accessible by so many. The proliferation of shopping malls, supermarkets and fast food restaurants has ensured this.

For this system to work financially, food marketers entice people to live high consumptive lifestyles.

Marketers know the way to get people to over consume is by appealing to their 'wants' rather than their 'needs'.

Can you remember the last time you heard a marketer tell you the key to your happiness is in 'consuming less'?

You're right. It never happens.

Food marketers use slick techniques to make women feel as if they can never have 'enough'.

This lifestyle of excess has been aided by marketing gimmicks. Common techniques include '2 for 1 offers', 'value meals' and portion upsizing.

It has also been spurred on by easy access to consumer credit.

The good news is that your body knows the truth.

It knows that more doesn't mean better. It also knows you can never fill an emotional void with fake food.

When you reconnect back to your body, it will let you know what you need to live a happy, healthy and inspired life.

Chapter summary.

There is so much misinformation about emotional eating. Like many things in life, it's not what you have been led to believe.

There is a lucrative 'corporate food fight' that has emerged over the past century. It works in direct opposition to the health aspirations of the emotional eater.

Becoming aware of this will help you to make better choices so you can *Heal Emotional Eating For Good.*

When I woke up to the bigger picture of emotional eating, I was able to start taking my power back. I stopped falling for all the marketing tricks designed to lure me into the consumption of fake food.

Instead I began seeking out things that could provide my body and soul with true nourishment.

I sought out companies who cared about the health of their customers. Those committed to making a positive contribution to the world, rather than only seeking profits.

You hold this same power.

You can build your awareness and seek out greater levels of truth for your self.

When you upgrade your routine food purchases you will be propelled along your healing journey.

This doesn't mean you need to become a 'perfect consumer' or fight against anything.

You also don't need to change your life overnight either.

Keep reminding yourself that healing is a journey.

And it all begins by taking baby steps...

Chapter Three – An Invitation to Start Your Healing Journey

"For me, it's not necessarily interesting to play a strong, fearless woman. It's interesting to play a woman who is terrified and then overcomes that fear. It's about the journey. Courage is not the absence of fear, it's overcoming it."

~ Natalie Dormer

Inspiring others to heal

"As soon as healing takes place, go out and heal somebody else."

~ Maya Angelou

A number of years after healing my body, I found myself teaching yoga on a traditional Greek Island.

Before arriving on the island I had hit an important transition point in my life. I had been heading in the wrong career direction for a while but felt uncertain about what I could do about it.

After my experience selling ice creams, I took on a series of sales and marketing roles. None of which worked out particularly well for me.

I struggled to find my place in the corporate world. I could see very little point to most of my assigned work projects. None of them seemed to make the world a better place.

I found myself in a cycle of working to 'pay the bills'. I would then quit in an attempt to claim back my freedom.

Despite having a degree in marketing, I had long suspected my true gifts lay elsewhere. I was daunted by the prospect of having to walk away from a career I was so heavily invested in.

I feared a career change would mean I had wasted all the years studying at university. Not to mention the ongoing financial costs of my student loan.

I was in a state of inner conflict.

My mind was telling me I needed to be cautious and come up with a practical plan of action.

My heart was telling me to let go of the past and focus upon the things that brought me true joy.

Morning meditation.

It was a Saturday morning and I had woken up with a busy mind.

I was in serious need of clarity. So I rolled out my yoga mat and did some gentle stretches. I then settled down for my morning meditation.

Both yoga and meditation had been key in helping me to heal my emotional eating and regain my health.

Sitting cross-legged on my yoga mat, I began to focus upon my breath. I gave myself full permission to let go of the pressure I had been putting on myself to come up with all the answers.

As my lungs inhaled and exhaled, I felt my tension begin to loosen and unwind. I followed my breath with a willingness to go wherever it wanted to take me.

This simple breath work helped me to drop into a much kinder and gentler space with myself. I soon began to feel my spirits lift.

Twenty minutes into my meditation, I felt the 'doors of my imagination' swing wide open.

I began to sense my dreams weren't wild fantasies to be ignored. I also considered my fears weren't as real as I had thought.

I had already learnt how to 'survive' by doing work I didn't enjoy.

I considered the time had come for me to 'thrive' by pursuing the things that brought my soul alive.

I let this profound prospect integrate into my being. And then a heart-expanding question dropped into my consciousness...

"What about applying for a job at a retreat centre?"

Wow... what a blissful idea! I felt my fears dissolve into bubbles of excitement and my whole body tingled with delight.

Perhaps this was the change of direction I had been searching for?

Open for opportunity.

After breakfast, I sat at my computer to research job opportunities. In my search, I stumbled upon an advertisement for a yoga teacher in the Greek Islands. It sounded like my dream job!

The retreat centre offered holistic holidays. They focused upon creative self-exploration within a supportive community environment.

I felt energised by the possibility. So I typed up my cover letter before I could have any second thoughts...

I then attached my resume, said a little prayer and hit the 'send' button.

***

For the Attention of the General Manager.

RE: Yoga Teaching Position in the Greek Islands.

I am a recently certified yoga teacher and massage therapist. I have an experiential understanding of the power of yoga to heal and a strong personal practice.

A decade ago, my body broke down and I was bed ridden for months. I was sick, tired and 60 pounds overweight.

My doctors wanted to treat my symptoms with experimental medication. Instead, I decided to immerse myself in the world of natural heath, healing and yoga.

By taking this path I was able to heal my chronic ailments, rebalance my body and release my excess weight. I also discovered a deep sense of peace and happiness within myself.

I would love the opportunity to share my passion for yoga and wellness with your guests. I am available for an immediate start.

Love Katrina

***

A week of waiting.

Summer was fast approaching. I assumed the retreat centre would be looking to hire a yoga teacher swiftly.

After an excruciating week of waiting, it dawned upon me they had decided to hire somebody else.

Although disappointed, I crossed my fingers and hoped another opportunity would emerge.

Much to my surprise, a week later I received an email from the General Manager of the retreat centre.

***

Dear Katrina

Thank you for applying for the yoga teaching position.

We have reviewed your application and would love to offer you the job.

We look forward to having you join our team!

Yours sincerely

The General Manager

***

I almost couldn't believe what I was reading.

My heart had guided me to step into the unknown and the Universe was responding.

I was thrilled to be given the opportunity. I emailed straight back saying I would love to accept the position.

I then started researching my flights to Greece…

Healing yoga and massage.

My job at the retreat centre was to teach the early morning yoga class. And in the afternoon I offered massage treatments.

In the corporate world, I spent much of my spare time studying personal development. I loved reading inspiring books and attending courses and workshops.

I completed trainings in yoga, massage, nutrition, coaching, hypnosis and other healing modalities.

Personal growth and self-discovery had long been passions of mine. It was wonderful to finally have the opportunity to use my skills professionally.

I held my daily yoga class on a platform with breathtaking views out towards the Aegean Sea.

The mornings were lovely and mild. There was enough sea breeze to keep everyone feeling relaxed and comfortable.

Most of my students were either new to yoga or out of practice.

So I focused upon keeping the classes accessible, light hearted and fun. This also helped me to find my natural flow as a teacher.

In the afternoons, I offered my massage treatments from my sun-filled therapy room.

When I trained as a massage therapist, we had been taught a specific sequence of strokes. This was to ensure each muscle group received sufficient coverage and to help us keep to time.

While I could see the benefits of this approach, I preferred to attune to the specific needs of my clients. To do this, I would ask my clients if they were experiencing any physical aches or pains within their body.

I then focused the bodywork upon the energetic blocks causing discomfort. At the end of the massage, I would also create space for my clients to provide feedback.

Some of them were too blissed out to speak which was great. I found most people enjoyed the extra support and used the opportunity to open up about their lives.

Most of my clients were women. They would often share the stresses they were experiencing back in the 'real world'. I was fascinated and eager to learn all I could.

If invited to do so, I would also offer my intuitive insights.

I soon noticed a connection between physical pain and mental and emotional patterns. I had noticed this on my healing journey and it was amazing to witness it in others as a practitioner.

Breakthrough Healing Sessions.

One morning after yoga, one of my students approached me and asked if I offered healing sessions?

I was already combining different healing modalities with my massage therapy work.

Without hesitation I responded, *"Yes of course"*.

"I've been struggling with my emotional eating" she said. *"After hearing your story, I had a strong feeling you might be able to offer me a fresh perspective"*.

The session we had together was amazing. She looked radiant afterwards, like a different woman.

She told me she had received a powerful *"breakthrough"* in the session.

She said she felt all this heaviness release from her body like a *"puff of smoke"*.

She then asked if she could share her experience with a couple of retreat friends. She was certain they would want to book sessions too.

And in that moment my *Breakthrough Healing Sessions* were born.

Creating my first flyer.

As my confidence in my work started to build, I decided to create a small flyer. This was so I could introduce my *Breakthrough Healing Sessions* to more people.

I wasn't attached to who responded to it.

I had faith that whoever needed to connect with my work would do so and step forward.

On the flyer I outlined my sessions and included a short story about my healing journey.

I hoped my students would find it inspiring to know their yoga teacher wasn't perfect. And that she had endured a health crisis, as well as lingering eating and weight challenges.

I also found the courage to share my 'before and after' photos.

There was a part of me that felt awkward and embarrassed.

I decided to ignore my inhibitions and revealed the photos anyway.

The flyer created a stir.

As soon as I placed it on the retreat notice board I was inundated with questions. People wanted to know how I had managed to overcome my weight problems and health challenges.

I even had one student pull me aside and ask *"Katrina is that before photo really of you or is it a picture of someone else?"*

The flyer removed any imaginary barrier that may have existed between my students and I.

It was incredible. It inspired many to book *Breakthrough Healing Sessions* with me.

Most wanted to release the past and transform their lives for the better.

Receiving feedback.

At first, the glowing testimony people gave me for my work was quite challenging to receive.

I was familiar with the criticism and political backstabbing of the corporate world. These encounters would often leave me in the nearest bathroom in floods of tears.

With time I was able to receive appreciation from my healing clients and yoga students.

The way I saw it, they were the ones who were being so brave.

My role was to inspire them to connect to their intuition and innate self-healing abilities.

I felt very privileged and humbled to hold this sacred healing space for other people.

I was delighted my life experience was beginning to serve a much bigger purpose.

I appreciated how much courage it takes for someone to look within and heal. And this made my work particularly meaningful.

People started booking *Breakthrough Healing Sessions* to work on all sorts of challenges.

This included emotional eating, weight loss and a host of other life issues.

Clients said the sessions helped them to release old mental and emotional patterns. Many were able to let go of limiting beliefs they had held onto for years.

Others shared they felt much lighter and more empowered to go after their dreams.

Before I knew it, I was booked solid for most of the summer...

Your invitation to start the healing journey

"Change is the essence of life. Be willing to surrender what you are for what you could become."

~ Reinhold Niebuhr

This book is your invitation to start your healing journey.

If you have been on your healing journey for a while, this book is an invitation to go even deeper.

The healing journey is all about releasing the beliefs, blocks, fears and stories holding you back.

I want you to create a life that is a full expression of who you are.

One that is meaningful to you and also fun and enjoyable to live.

Your emotional eating is a signal there is healing work to be done.

As you start to release the things that are not true for you, your emotional eating will subside.

You will also find that your mind, body and emotions will start to rebalance.

Now you might think it seems a little unusual to have someone else invite you to look inside and heal?

And I'd have to agree with you.

It's not an everyday occurrence!

It would be nice to think we could let go of the past and become the best version of ourselves all on our own.

In my experience, we all need a little inspiration, guidance and support from the Universe.

Challenges are healing invitations in disguise.

On my own journey I have received many different invitations to heal various aspects of my life.

Some of the healing invitations came disguised as challenges like:

- Emotional eating.
- Chronic fatigue and adrenal exhaustion.
- Asthma, eczema and other health conditions.
- Persistent weight challenges.
- University studies I wasn't inspired by.
- Friendships without common interests or values.
- Relationships that weren't right for me.
- Financial pressures and debt burdens.
- Jobs I felt frustrated and stuck in.

By seeing my challenges as invitations to heal, I have been able to transform my life in miraculous ways.

Each of these healing invitations created the opportunity for me to understand who I am. And what I stand for in this world.

These invitations enabled me to heal and rebalance my body.

They also inspired me to lose 60 pounds, travel the world, express myself, get paid for work I love and marry my soul mate.

Each healing invitation I received taught me how to listen to and trust my intuition.

It also helped me to have the courage to release all the things I had outgrown.

These invitations helped me to turn down the volume on the voices on the outside. Many of which were well meaning.

As I gained a better understanding of what was true and meaningful for me, I was able to re-create my life.

An invitation to start your healing journey.

The invitation to heal, regardless of the form it arrives in, is a very beautiful and sacred thing.

I love to get invited to things. Especially the things I know have the ability to transform my life for the better. It creates feelings of excitement, possibility and a sense of adventure inside of me.

And this is why I want to invite you to start your own healing journey. So you too can *Heal Emotional Eating For Good.*

I am making this invitation on behalf of you and your highest potential.

This invitation is an open one and comes without conditions.

There is no RSVP date.

You don't need to respond if you don't want to. Your response doesn't make you a good or bad person.

The only reason to respond to this invitation is if you know in your heart you are ready to start.

Healing is not a race. It is not a sport or some kind of competition. It's not something you can use to compare yourself to others.

You won't be receiving any medals, ribbons or trophies for going on this journey. There are no certificates to be had. No diplomas, degrees or even doctorates. Nor are there any special commendations.

This journey is not likely to impress or win the approval of your family, friends or co-workers.

That is unless they have already been on their own journey of self-discovery.

The only reason to accept this invitation is if you feel moved to.

Choose this path if you want to learn more about yourself and what is possible for you in this lifetime.

Connecting with your true self.

The healing journey is a way to discover your true nature and live by your deepest values.

This journey is a personal one and is of great importance to the evolution of your soul. It is a journey that only you can walk for yourself. No one else can do it for you.

On this journey you have the opportunity to heal and release all the things that are no longer serving you.

This includes old thoughts, feelings and behaviours you have outgrown. You can heal and release painful memories, regrets, disappointments, frustrations and even trauma.

It also includes releasing possessions you feel weighed down by.

Old entanglements can be burdensome to hold on to.

The key is to either transform them into something that serves you or lovingly release them.

On the healing journey you get to learn how to build a kind and loving relationship with your self.

You get to recognise and appreciate the things that make you beautiful and unique.

To make progress on my own healing journey, I chose to make my courage bigger than my fears.

Now this may sound a little scary at first, particularly if it is not something you are familiar with.

Rest assured this is something that becomes easier with time.

Cultivating courage is like a building a muscle. When you neglect your 'courage muscles' they will atrophy.

When you engage them, they will strengthen.

Connecting with others.

Even though this is a personal journey, there will be many new people for you to meet along the way.

There will be fellow travellers, guides and mentors who can assist and inspire you.

On this journey it is important you place yourself in supportive surroundings.

Choose environments that inspire you to be true to yourself and help you create the life you want.

This includes the places you live, work and socialise in.

On this journey, you don't need to conform to the rules and expectations of others.

Or seek permission from anyone else.

You already have full permission to follow your heart, hopes and highest aspirations.

On the healing journey you also get to explore the impact others have had upon your life.

You get to give thanks for the lessons they have given you and also forgive them for any harm they may have caused.

On this journey you also get to look within and forgive yourself.

This includes being brave enough to witness the hidden parts of you that you would prefer to turn away from.

Especially the parts that make you feel embarrassed, ashamed, guilty and unworthy.

As hard as it may seem now, please know these parts are worthy of your recognition, acceptance and love.

Getting started on your healing journey.

You will know within yourself when you are ready to begin your healing journey.

The only place you can start this journey is from where you are.

You don't need any special talents or abilities to get started. Just a willingness to take the next step as it presents itself.

My invitation to start the healing journey came disguised as a body breakdown.

As hard as this invitation was for me to receive, it changed the course of my life forever. It is something I will always be grateful for.

When I discovered the healing journey, I realised it was the path I had been searching for.

Your emotional eating is a sacred invitation to become the best version of your self.

When you attune to it, this powerful feedback mechanism will let you know when you are either 'on' or 'off' course.

It will offer you incredible insights about your life and also reveal the next layer of healing work to be done.

If you allow it, your emotional eating will become your very own 'spiritual compass'. You can use it to guide you as you travel along your healing journey.

All you need to do is create space and allow it to reveal its' precious wisdom to you.

Trust it will give you everything you need to heal and rebalance your body, mind and spirit.

This is your life and it is up to you to keep moving this adventure forward. Allow yourself to move in a direction that is inspiring and meaningful to you.

Chapter summary.

By the end of my first season in the Greek Islands, it was clear that I could never work in an office again.

The feedback from my yoga students and healing clients let me know I was headed in the right direction.

I was invited back to the retreat centre the following season. This one invitation gave me the chance to share and develop my healing work.

Soon other retreat centres around the world began inviting me to share my yoga and healing work.

This gave me the confidence to run my own *Yoga and Healing Retreats.*

This little Greek Island was so special to me that my husband and I married there.

We exchanged our vows as the sun set over the Aegean Sea in a simple and beautifully romantic ceremony.

It was one of the most treasured moments of my life.

In a surprising twist, I can also share my marketing studies were not in vain as I had feared.

When I started my own business, I came to appreciate how valuable these skills are. Particularly when they are dedicated towards the service of others.

On this journey I've learnt that none of our experiences are wasted.

Everything we encounter, no matter how difficult, is here to teach us something.

And all we need to do is be willing to accept the gift.

Chapter Four – The Inner World of Emotional Eating

"Our inner guidance comes to us through our feelings and body wisdom first, not through intellectual understanding."

~ Christiane Northrup, M.D.

Emotional eating is not the real problem

"All forms of self-defeating behavior are unseen and unconscious, which is why their existence is denied."

~ Vernon Howard

Diane booked a series of *Breakthrough Healing Sessions* with me.[4]

She worked in a high-pressure corporate environment.

Diane had come to a point in her life where she felt trapped in a desperate cycle.   What she wanted most was to reconnect with her passion for life.

"I just feel so exhausted that I'm close to giving up…" she said. *"To be honest, I've been feeling this way for a long time now."*

Diane shared she used to have high levels of energy and enthusiasm for life.

Now she felt as if she was *"going through the motions"*.

Her home life was also challenging.

She was a mother to two young children and was the family's main breadwinner.

She held a lot of repressed anger towards her husband. She resented their shared predicament and they would often argue with each other.

Diane said it was like she was living *"someone else's life"* and she felt powerless to do anything about it.

---

[4] Please note client names and details have been changed throughout this book.

Adding to her stress levels was the fact she hated looking at herself in the mirror.

She said all her clothes felt *"too tight"* on her and she felt *"disconnected from her body"*.

The stress of her life was causing her to live from her head whilst trying to silence her body with food.

Diane told me her comfort food of choice was chocolate ice cream.

She said it wasn't uncommon for her to eat a whole tub in front of the television over the course of an evening.

She would often say to herself *"Diane, eat the ice cream now and deal with the problem tomorrow"*.

Like many women, she found she didn't have time to devote to her personal wellbeing the following day.

Having the courage to move forward.

In our initial session, I encouraged Diane to focus upon her breath.

As we sat breathing together I could feel her reconnect with her body's natural intelligence.

I shared with her that when mind and body are disconnected it is difficult to find balance and flow in life.

Once Diane was a little more relaxed, I revealed that emotional eating was a stress response.

Because of this she didn't need to try and control her emotional eating.

Instead what we needed to do was look at ways of reducing her mental, emotional and physical stress load.

"You're right about my high stress levels…" she said. *"It's no wonder I haven't had any luck trying to control my cravings…"*

How I start a Breakthrough Healing Session.

Over the years, I have conducted *Breakthrough Healing Sessions* with hundreds of women like Diane.

At the start of a healing session, I ask clients what they would like to work on.

Most say they want to work on whatever they think their problem is.

For example a client might say they want to work on their 'emotional eating' or 'weight problem'.

This is an excellent starting point.

But what I have found is that the problem my clients 'think' they have is usually not the 'real problem'.

I asked Diane about the types of things she had done to try and 'solve' her emotional eating.

She said she had spent *"many thousands of dollars"* in an attempt to control her cravings and lose weight.

"I've tried everything Katrina... Really I have... and nothing seems to work for me..." she said.

Diane ran through all the different things she had attempted over the years.

This included buying the latest diet books, low calorie meals and exercise machines.

"Katrina, I've spent so many years trying to fix my emotional eating it's become insufferable..." she said.

"I don't understand it. I'm an intelligent woman. I'm great at my job. And I'm successful in other areas of my life..."

"So why is it I can't seem to stop my emotional eating?"

When I hear questions like this, I totally get it.

I know exactly how confusing and frustrating it can be.

It took me many years to make any kind of sense out of my own emotional eating patterns.

And finally break free of the dieting cycle.

As with most things, not understanding the problem makes it hard to find the right solution.

"Diane the reason why most diet products fail is because they focus on the symptoms of our emotional eating..." I said. *"Rather than address the underlying root cause..."*

"To heal I needed to move beyond thinking my emotional eating was the problem..."

"I had to find the courage to look inside and identify what was driving my emotional eating... By being willing to look within I was able to access deeper layers of personal truth..."

My healing journey called me to get honest about the things I wanted. It also invited me to build awareness of the things causing me stress and emotional pain.

I started this process by paying attention to my innermost thoughts and feelings.

I also began attuning to my body and the archive of wisdom it contains. And I learnt how to take better care of it.

The root causes of our emotional eating can take time and patience to uncover. This is because they are largely unconscious.

As any gardener will tell you, if you want to remove weeds from your garden, you have to pull them out from the root.

If you only pull the stem, the weed will keep growing back bigger and stronger...

My annual newsletter survey.

Each year I send out a survey to my newsletter subscribers. I do this to find out about the challenges confronting women in their daily lives. Here's a sample of recent responses:

"I'm so fed up! I can't go on like this any longer..."

"I feel like I really need some room to breathe..."

"I've tried everything, but nothing seems to work. I feel like I'm missing something... I just want to feel peaceful."

"I'm sick and tired of trying to be the perfect mother, wife and home maker... I feel so empty and low."

"I'd cry but to be honest, I just don't have time."

"I'm terribly exhausted. I've got nothing left to give. I feel like I'm on the verge of breakdown..."

"I'm either one way or the other. I'm all good and healthy or if I'm not, I'm eating really badly, not exercising and just feeling terrible."

"I've given up smoking (and chewing tobacco). But now I have these constant cravings for coffee, sugar and sweets all the time."

"I'm so worried about money. I don't have enough to pay my bills. Even if I do manage to pay them, I start worrying about how I'll pay them next month. It's a constant and never-ending worry for me."

"Even though I have people in my life, I still feel so alone."

"If I was the crying type, I'd be on the floor bawling my eyes out..."

"I dream of quietness, being in nature and having some time for me..."

"I'd love to create and do something meaningful with my life..."

"I want to be true to myself and feel happy. Is that too much to ask?"

We all have our own unique relationship to stress.

Which survey responses do you relate to?

I am always moved by the responses I receive. They often remind me of the challenges I have had to confront and work through in my life.

They also highlight the unprecedented levels of stress women are under today.

Have you ever felt pressure to be the perfect daughter, girlfriend, lover, or spouse? I know I have at different times in my life.

Society imposes all kinds of expectations and burdens upon women. It is important to build awareness of the stress placed upon us from the outside world.

We also need to be aware of the stress we create within ourselves.

We all have our own unique way of dealing with stress. As well as individual stress tolerance levels too.

What is stressful for one woman may not be stressful to another.

There is no need to compare your ability to cope with stress to anyone else.

Some women thrive on a lot of stress, whereas others may only be able to contend with small amounts.

Emotional eating is a signal you are reaching a limit of how much stress you can deal with in the moment.

It's important to observe the things that cause you stress.

You can release stress by experimenting with different healing tools.

When you release stress, anxiety and overwhelm, you create space for something new.

Is all stress bad?

One thing I like to share with my clients is that there are two types of stress: *'good stress'* and *'bad stress'*.

My focus with clients is to help them optimise the positive effects of good stress. And minimise the negative effects of bad stress.

So what exactly is good stress?

Good stress gives you energy, vitality and flow in your life. It supports you to act in alignment with your highest values and aspirations, as well as your dreams. It also helps you to live a life you love and achieve the things most important to you.

Good stress is healthy for your body, mind and spirit. It plays an important role in helping you to realise your true potential.

It can help you strive for deadlines. Like working to finish an important project or making a special effort for a social function.

Once the deadline or event has passed, our lives return to normal and our stress levels rebalance.

Bad stress robs you of your energy, rhythm and natural flow. It can create chronic anxiety and overwhelm that's hard to recover from. It can also create a sense there is no way out of a situation.

Bad stress can create forms of self-sabotaging behaviour such as resistance and procrastination. It can also result in the need to use a coping strategy like emotional eating.

Bad stress tends to build up gradually making it hard to detect. If left unaddressed, it can lead to adverse consequences. Such as a physical breakdown as was the case for me.

* Please note: When I am discussing the stress that causes emotional eating throughout the book, I am referring to 'bad stress'.

Emotional eating is a coping strategy

"Nothing ever goes away until it has taught us what we need to know."

~ Pema Chödrön

In *Losing Weight is a Healing Journey* I defined emotional eating as

"a scenario where food is used to manage, regulate and even medicate uncomfortable feelings on a regular or habitual basis".

Or in other words, emotional eating is a 'coping strategy'.

A coping strategy enables a person to carry on attending to their everyday demands. This is without having to address deeper life issues or concerns. These concerns can include unhealed experiences of the past or fear and anxiety about the future.

Emotional eating is not an attempt to resolve stressful thoughts and feelings. But rather, a way to soothe, pacify and placate them.

The trouble with coping strategies is they don't address the real problem. As a result, they can never provide a permanent solution.

A coping strategy can yield temporary relief and distraction from the pain, hurt and stress you may be experiencing in your life. Thus helping you to feel better in the moment.

Once the temporal effects have worn off, you will end up feeling worse.

This is because the underlying cause of stress and overwhelm remains unaddressed and unresolved.

Although emotional eating is a common coping strategy for many women, it is by no means the only one.

Other coping strategies include excessive shopping, exercise, television, sex, smoking, alcohol, drugs, work, gossip and even drama.

Does using a coping strategy make you a bad person?

Despite what the dieting industry would have you believe, you are not a bad person for using emotional eating to deal with stress.

Coping strategies are nothing to be ashamed of. They don't mean you are weak willed or lacking in self-discipline. It took me a while to work this out for myself.

I want you to know there is a time and place for coping strategies.

Life is messy. And coping strategies can provide women with temporary emotional and psychological benefits. Particularly when they are unable to resolve stressful circumstances in the moment. I was an emotional eater for nearly a decade. And for a while it did help to make me feel better.

Where coping strategies turn problematic is when they become our default approach to life. Or in other words, when a 'short-term solution' turns into a 'long-term strategy'.

If the underlying emotional stress is left unaddressed, it can have downstream consequences.

Emotional eating can affect your physical wellbeing. It can cause bloating, weight gain, sleep issues and other imbalances.

Emotional eating can also affect the quality of your inner wellbeing.

It can create feelings of guilt, self-attack and the desire for self-punishment. These stressful feelings can create the conditions for further food binging episodes. Emotional eating can morph into a vicious cycle that strengthens and reinforces itself.

With the benefit of hindsight I was able to see my emotional eating had very little to do with food.

My downfall was I didn't have the awareness or healing tools to deal with my stress in a more empowering way.

When I knew better, I was able to transform my life for the better.

Everyone is fighting some kind of battle.

I have run *Breakthrough Healing Sessions* with people from all walks of life. This includes many successful celebrity and high net worth clients.

I have come to see first hand that each of us is fighting some kind of battle.

If your life is feeling difficult at the moment, you are not alone.

We all have unique challenges to confront and work through in this lifetime.

People who experience success in one area of life can often face big challenges in others.

One thing that has become clear to me from doing my healing work is that we are all doing the best we can.

This is especially true when you take into account someone's individual nature, awareness levels and life story.

Now life wouldn't be much fun if we were only given challenges without a way of resolving them right?

Each of us have been given special talents to triumph over our tribulations.

These natural talents and abilities await your recognition, cultivation and development.

The trouble for most is we remain asleep to the power we have residing dormant within us.

Your emotional eating is a way for you to discover your innate gifts and natural talents.

You can use these abilities to rise above your challenges and become the very best person you can be.

The profit motive of the dieting industry.

The dieting industry would like to distract you from the inner power residing within you.

It does this by convincing women to give their attention to the latest dieting trends and fads.

And this is despite the fact the dieting model has an accepted failure rate of 95%.

The dieting industry wants you to believe you have to control your emotional eating. They encourage you to focus on calorie counting, portion control and food restriction.

I spent a good deal of my teenage years trying to solve my 'weight problem' using these methodologies.

Each time a new diet would appear I would become hopeful about the prospect of my life changing for the better.

Of course my end results were always disappointing.

As I attempted each new diet, it wouldn't take long for my emotional eating to flare up.

Dieting would trigger uncomfortable feelings inside me. Without providing any healing tools to address and release them.

I had no idea how to use these feelings to transform my life. Instead I sought relief from my feelings through my favourite comfort foods.

Trying to control my emotional eating through dieting had the opposite effect to what I intended.

Not only did I gain far more weight than I ever lost, it also stripped me of my courage, confidence and self-esteem.

By the time my body broke down, I'd almost given up on the idea of ever being able to lose weight. Or reign in my emotional eating.

I thought there was something wrong with me.

My dieting failures convinced me there must be something wrong with me.

This led me to go on a relentless search to find out why I was so 'bad' at dieting.

After enduring years of shame, I discovered my dieting story was a similar story shared by many women.

The sad reality is most women fail at dieting and gain more weight than they lose.

Perhaps this has been true in your experience too?

The thing I began to recognise is the reason why diets fail is because they have been 'designed to fail'.

The dieting industry has no interest in helping you understand your inner most thoughts and feelings.

It ignores the root cause of emotional eating and as a consequence the miraculous nature of the solution.

It has no incentive in liberating its customer base from their weight concerns. And it certainly doesn't want you to *Heal Emotional Eating For Good.*

The last thing this multi-billion dollar industry wants to do is put itself out of business.

What they are interested in is getting women to buy into the 'dieting model' so they can profit from us forever.

The dieting industry is well aware the money is in keeping women sick, tired and overweight. It's not in helping them to become healthy, happy and free.

And once they've got you hooked, they have endless things to sell you to keep you distracted from the truth.

You could waste lifetimes wading through their packaged meals, diet soft drinks and exercise machines. And still be no further along in your journey.

Glossy women's magazines and other forms of mainstream media add to the confusion.

They publish contradictory dieting information to keep women feeling disorientated, frustrated and stuck.

They generate massive advertising revenues from spreading lies and deception. They design ad campaigns to keep women in a perpetual state of guilt and shame around their bodies.

They make you feel as if the only way you can change your life is by consuming the products they advertise.

They sell the idea that happiness is 'an outside job'. All you need is the right clothes, shoes, make up, hairstyle, perfume, jewelry, car, house and lover. And then your life will be amazing.

The truth is that true fulfillment has and always will be 'an inside job'.

It is your inner world that creates your experience of the outer world and not the other way around.

If you want to heal, you must see this haze of misinformation and confusion for what it is.

You are a magnificent creation.

You do not have to believe anyone that tries to convince you otherwise.

Take back your power from the institutions that profit from your struggle.

You can then reinvest that energy into healing yourself and pursuing your dreams.

And when you do, your life will transform forever…

Emotional eating has costs and pay-offs

"Eating crappy food isn't a reward - it's a punishment."

~ Drew Carey

Many women book *Breakthrough Healing Sessions* with me when their 'coping strategies' stop working.

Or when the cost of their emotional eating strategy starts to outweigh the pay-offs.

The **cost** of a coping strategy is the pain, suffering and lost opportunities it creates in your life. Although the costs start out low, they tend to accumulate over time.

The **pay-off** of a coping strategy is the benefit it gives you. The pay-off may feel significant in the beginning but the effects tend to lesson over time.

The reason we use coping strategies is because the perceived pay-offs outweigh the perceived costs.

When a coping strategy adds more pain than it relieves, transformation becomes possible.

Most emotional eaters are unaware of the costs and pay-offs of their coping strategy.

In my case, it took a big shock for me to start paying closer attention.

You do not need to hit rock bottom in order to heal.

You can begin to reduce the stress driving your emotional eating right now.

A great way to start is by building your awareness of the hidden costs and pay-offs that underpin your emotional eating...

The costs and pay-offs of my emotional eating.

When I started on the path of emotional eating as a young teenager I was in a pretty healthy place. I was able to manage my emotions with food without any serious physical consequences.

At this innocent starting point, the 'pay-offs' of my emotional eating were high and the 'costs' were low.

They were the perfect conditions for my food addiction to form and develop unnoticed.

With the passing of time, my body began to show signs of moving out of balance and I started gaining weight.

Soon the kids at school started making fun of me behind my back.

Even my well-meaning grandfather, pulled me aside one day to tell me I was getting *"chubby"*.

It wasn't long before I became a young woman who was shy, self-conscious and ashamed of her body.

As my teenage years progressed, I started to turn to food whenever I was feeling sad or lonely.

The good feelings I received from my emotional eating outweighed the costs. So I saw no compelling reason to do anything different.

After the incident with Jake, my emotional eating became the glue that held my life together. And then one day it stopped working.

When my body broke down it was clear I could no longer walk the path I was on. Being bed ridden for months and being spoon-fed by my mother, was all the proof I needed to confirm this.

The costs of my emotional eating had finally exceeded the pay-offs.

The time had come for me to find the courage to move in a new direction or risk even more dire heath consequences.

My cost and pay-off analysis.

Before I could start changing my life, I needed to have a deeper understanding of my emotional eating.

I had been studying about the concept of costs and pay-offs in my marketing degree. I decided to see if I could apply the same approach to assess my emotional eating…

While I was in my sick bed, I took out a notebook and began to journal the costs and pay-offs of my predicament.

Some of the costs I experienced from emotional eating included:

- Loss of self confidence, self esteem and self worth
- Increased feelings of lethargy and depression
- Weight gain of over 60 pounds
- Chronic fatigue and adrenal exhaustion
- Self attack after emotional eating episodes
- Not feeling good enough
- Feeling sick and tired
- Lack of energy to do the things I wanted to do
- A lack of depth and intimacy in my friendships

Some of the pay-offs I experienced from emotional eating included:

- Instant gratification that came from eating whatever I wanted
- Not having to change my behaviour or do something different
- Not having to deal with my true feelings
- Not having to take responsibility for my thoughts and beliefs
- Not having to risk sharing my pain with other people
- Not having to get honest with myself
- Not having to take responsibility for my health
- Not having to listen and attune to my body's needs
- Being able to soothe my uncomfortable feelings with food
- Feeling as if the rules didn't apply to me
- Confirmation of my belief I wasn't good enough

Helping Diane get clear on her costs and pay-offs.

I shared what I had learnt about costs and pay-offs with Diane.

I have found most clients are aware of the costs of their emotional eating. But are unaware of the pay-offs.

Diane and I worked through the exercise together. I asked her to close her eyes to see if she could connect with the costs of her emotional eating strategy.

Diane reeled off the following costs...

- She felt out of control and ashamed of herself
- Her emotional eating was draining her life force energy
- It was making her body feel fat and bloated
- It was making her feel hopeless and unhappy with her life
- It was expensive to feed her addictions
- She felt like she wasn't being a good example to her children
- She was sabotaging her happiness at home and at work
- She felt depleted and unsure of what to do about it

Diane found the second part of the exercise a little more difficult. She had to challenge herself to find her emotional eating pay-offs.

Here are the payoffs that she shared…

- She could use food to try and make herself feel better
- She didn't have to do anything different
- She didn't have to take responsibility for her health
- She didn't have to address her work related stress
- She didn't have to address her relationship with herself
- She didn't have to make any changes in her life
- She could indulge herself whenever she liked
- She had the feeling she was getting what she deserved
- She had a good reason to feel angry all the time
- She was able to blame her husband for their situation
- She was able to criticise herself like her parents did

Exercise: Emotional eating cost and pay-off worksheet.

List the costs and pay-offs of your emotional eating below.

a) Make a list of the costs of your emotional eating...

| |
| |
| |
| |
| |
| |
| |
| |

b) Make a list of the pay-offs of your emotional eating…

| |
| |
| |
| |
| |
| |
| |
| |

Chapter summary.

Emotional eating is not the real problem. This is why it cannot be resolved through willpower or by trying to control your food intake.

Emotional eating is a call for you to look inwards and start paying attention to your life. It is a call to follow your dreams and be true to yourself.

Healing happens when you listen to your cravings and allow them to give you feedback about your life. Give yourself permission to feel your feelings, rather than feed them.

Instead of using food to soothe and comfort, ask yourself questions like:

- What am I truly hungry for?
- What am I really craving?
- What am I ready to do differently?

With time you will recognise the stressful thoughts and feelings at the root of your emotional eating.

Instead of using fake food as a coping strategy, you can choose to use healing tools instead.

Emotional eating has both costs and pay-offs.

When the pay-offs are more than the costs your emotional eating will continue.

When the costs of emotional eating outweigh the pay-offs, it becomes possible to *Heal Emotional Eating For Good.*

Your emotional eating is a gift and it is here to teach you something important.

Look upon it as a place you are passing through on your healing journey and not as your final destination.

PHASE 2:

Emotional Healing

Chapter Five – Choose to Heal

"You have resources yet to be unleashed. Make bold, courageous choices.   Live as though you have the power to change the world - because you do."

~ Caroline Myss

Make the choice to heal

"The most important choice is the decision to heal; all else follows."

~ Wanda Buckner

I was sick. That much was clear.

What remained uncertain was whether I would be able to do anything about it.

I was sitting on a plastic blue chair next to my mother in the waiting room of my local medical centre.

I had a sinking feeling in the pit of my stomach.

The room smelt as if it was peppered with disinfectant. The warm air that wafted out of the gas heater was catching the back of my throat.

As a child riddled with allergies and illness, I had spent many hours in that waiting room staring at the clock.

Tick tock.

My mother had booked an appointment with my doctor to discuss my test results.

I gazed around the fluorescently lit room. It didn't appear to be the kind of place you would visit voluntarily in the search of health and happiness.

The coffee table in the centre of the room had out-of-date gossip magazines strewn all over it.

The walls were plastered with posters imploring flu jabs, blood thinners and measles inoculations.

And the floors were covered in grey carpet tiles that frayed in the high traffic areas.

To my right a middle-aged woman coughed and spluttered as she tried to keep her bronchitis all to herself.

To my left, a little boy sat sniffling as his mother comforted him.

An elderly man shuffled his way into the room with the aid of his walking frame. Each step he took appeared as if it might be his last.

The assembled characters all reflected something about the wretchedness of my predicament.

The doctor entered the room in a self-assured fashion.

She was wearing a crisply pressed lab coat over her civilian clothes and her hair was pulled back tight in a bun. Adding to her steely façade was a stethoscope that ornamented her slender neck.

She glanced at the manila folder she was carrying in her hands. With an upward inflection she called my name *"Katrina?"*

My mother helped me to my feet. We exchanged greetings and then followed her into the consultation room.

She invited us to take a seat. She then sat down behind her white laminate desk and started reviewing my test results.

The doctor rested her spectacles on the tip of her nose as she examined the report.

She said it was difficult to pinpoint exactly what was wrong with me. And she recommended treating my symptoms with a course of experimental medication.

When I enquired about how long I would need to be on medication for, she replied *"possibly for life."*

I listened in disbelief.

Surely this couldn't be happening to me...

As much as I respected my doctor's opinion, my intuition said *"No! There has to be another way..."*

I had just turned 20 years old. It seemed a little premature for anyone to be making predictions about how the rest of my life would unfold.

I imagined what it would be like spending my life worrying about pills and prescriptions.

I had spent much of my youth on various kinds of tablets, creams and inhalers. I used them to combat my chronic asthma, eczema and allergies.

The last thing I wanted was to be given a life sentence on pharmaceuticals.

I thought there had to be natural treatment options available without the risk of side effects.

I thanked my doctor for sharing her findings. I told her I would need some time to consider my next steps.

A decision of this size had the ability to affect my entire life. I didn't want to commit to something within the walls of that consultation room I would later regret.

My mother and I drove home from the doctor's surgery in silence. I felt too upset to speak and asked if we could save the discussion for when my father returned home from work.

I locked myself in my bedroom for the rest of the afternoon. I needed some time to process what my doctor had said and to be with my innermost feelings.

I was scared about having to discuss my doctor's recommendations with my parents.

Would they give me the space to make my own decision?

Or, would they side with my doctor and insist that I take the medication?

Taking time to get honest with myself.

For the next few hours my mind spun with a random array of thoughts...

"I can't keep living like this!"

"I'm sick and tired of being sick and tired."

"Something has to shift."

"I want to change the circumstances of my life."

"Things can never go back to the way they have been."

"This time is different."

"I'm ready to make some changes."

"I don't want to take the medication."

"I can choose to eat foods that are better for me."

"I know I don't have all the answers."

"I don't know anything about healing."

"Maybe I can learn how to heal myself?"

"My health is my responsibility."

"No one can tell me how to live my life... This is my body."

"I can take better care of myself... I know I can."

"I am willing to make mistakes and learn as I go along."

"I am willing to stretch and grow."

"I am ready to start healing my life."

Facing the music.

The few hours locked away in my bedroom were precious. It gave me the opportunity to get clear about what I was going to say to my parents. It also helped me contemplate how I wanted to live my life.

Up until that point, I had been so focused upon pleasing everyone else. I hadn't considered the importance of my happiness.

So what did I want? Now that was a big question to ask.

I knew I wanted to feel happy and whole within myself. I wanted to break free from my emotional eating patterns and restore my health.

I wanted my stomach, hips and thighs to shrink and for the excess weight around my face, neck, chest and arms to melt away. I wanted to feel strong in my body and free to live my life as I saw fit.

I wanted to become a powerful woman in charge of her own destiny. I couldn't stand the thought of living out the rest of my life as a victim.

I was certain I didn't want to take the medication. In fact I wanted to liberate myself from the medical world forever.

Creating the space to listen to the wisdom of my heart was powerful. I felt something surge within me.

This feeling gave me the courage and confidence to move beyond my fears and perceived limits.

Later that evening I sat down with my parents and took a deep breath.

"Mum... Dad... I'm not going to take the medication."

"Are you sure love?" my mother asked.

"Yes I'm sure Mum. I want to heal myself naturally..."

It was amazing to hear the words come out of my mouth.

I had finally made the choice to heal. And it felt exhilarating...

Getting started on the healing journey.

One of the most common questions I receive from women is *"How do I get started on the healing journey?"*

I would have liked to have known the answer to this myself, when I was struggling with emotional eating.

Phase 1 is a very necessary and important part of the healing journey.

It's a phase of innocence, inexperience and the eventual mishaps.

In Phase 1, I tried to control my emotional eating through dieting. When I did this my results were always disappointing.

Sooner or later my willpower would wane and I would return back to my old habits, frustrated and none the wiser.

I was making decisions based upon my old patterns and ways of thinking. What I needed was to gain a new level of knowledge and awareness that could transform my life.

To move myself out of Phase 1, I had to make the choice to heal.

This clarity came to me after my body broke down and I was suffering in a 'world of pain'.

Sitting with the daunting prospect of having to take medication for the rest of my life shook me awake. It activated something inside of me.

It made me look at my lifestyle and how I had been living.

I was sick of my old eating habits and coping strategies. And my body had given me a very clear 'warning shot' that it was in trouble.

I didn't want to lose control over my body. I realised I had to finally take responsibility for my life.

I committed to becoming more aware of the choices I was making. I wanted to have a deeper understanding of the impact they were having upon my health and wellbeing.

Choosing to heal.

Albert Einstein said insanity was *"doing the same thing over and over again and expecting different results."*

When you make the choice to heal, you move out of Phase 1 of the healing journey and begin Phase 2.

Phase 2 on the healing journey is about cleaning up your past.

It's also about imagining new possibilities for your future. Moving into this phase only becomes necessary once you have something to heal.

Making a choice means to select one option over all others. It means you are ready to do something different and are willing to change the course of your destiny.

Making the choice to heal gives you the ability to move your life force energy in the direction you want. Rather than have it directed by others.

Most women begin Phase 2 in some form of physical, mental or emotional pain. Although it was hard for me to go through at the time, I can now see that my pain was a gift.

When I had attempted to make changes in the past, I had always retreated back to what was comfortable.

It was so liberating for me to discover I could create space for new possibilities to emerge in my life. And for me to realise I didn't have to go back to my old unconscious eating habits, patterns and conditioning.

I held the power to choose my thoughts, feelings and actions for myself.

I could also choose what foods to put inside my body and decide whether to take medication.

When you make the choice to heal your emotional eating, you step onto the path of long-term success.

Exercise: Signs you are ready to heal your emotional eating.

The healing journey commences the moment you choose to heal and change your life for the better.

Below is a list of signs you are ready to start your healing journey.

Signs you are ready to start your healing journey.	Yes / No
I am ready to change.	
I am ready to release the pain of my past.	
I am willing to ask for support.	
I am willing to make my health and healing a priority.	
I am willing to connect with the wisdom of my body.	
I am willing to embrace new thoughts and ideas.	
I am willing to eat healing foods.	
I am willing to invest time and energy into healing.	
I am willing to put myself first.	
I am willing to increase my levels of self care.	
I am willing to prioritise my happiness.	
I am willing to do the things that work.	
I am willing to look within.	
I am willing to accept responsibility for my health.	
I am willing to be courageous.	
I have made the choice to heal.	

Set a healing intention

"Every journey begins with the first step of articulating the intention, and then becoming the intention."

~ Bryant McGill

Once you have made the choice to heal your emotional eating, the next thing is to set your 'healing intention'.

A **healing intention** will guide you to heal and release all the things that are no longer serving you.

It will support you to rise above your emotional eating and open to your true destiny.

A healing intention is first formed in your mind and felt in your heart. It is then activated through the use of your will.

Healing intentions allow you to create clarity around what is most important to you.

They also mobilise your resourcefulness to take inspired action.

It will provide you with a point of focus so you can live with purpose and passion.

A good healing intention will help you to overcome any challenge you encounter on your healing journey.

It will also provide you with the courage to follow your intuition and live your highest potential.

Your intention brings the qualities of your desired end result into the present moment.

It allows you to connect with all the good feelings you hope to experience in the future right now.

Let your healing intentions guide you.

Your healing intention helps you to make better decisions by guiding you towards what you say 'yes' and 'no' to.

Setting a healing intention will assist you to clarify who you are and what you stand for in this world. It will help bring your greatest hopes and aspirations to life.

A good intention is one that requires you to grow into the person you are capable of becoming.

Your healing intention is something you need to cultivate and nurture into existence.

It is the seed of your potential and what is possible for you.

Once a seed is planted it needs adequate water, nutrients and sunshine to grow into its full glory.

Creating a healing intention gave me the inspiration to keep moving forward. Particularly when I was feeling uncertain, confused or afraid.

It enabled me to bring my attention back to my vision of what was possible.

It also connected me to the things that brought me joy and happiness.

My healing intention was the golden flame that lit me from within and illuminated my path.

It gave me the courage to address the stress that had been driving my emotional eating.

It also gave me the necessary power and strength to be myself and to release the things I had outgrown. You too hold this power.

Set your healing intention.

Let it be the compass that guides you along your healing journey.

How I use healing intentions in my yoga classes.

When I teach yoga, I like to create space for my students to become active participants in their own experience.

To achieve this, I encourage them to attune to the wisdom held within their bodies.

Some days the body will be happy and willing to experience a more dynamic yoga practice.

Other days it may prefer a more restorative class.

I start each one of my yoga classes by saying, *"Let your body be your teacher and allow me to be your guide."*

Once my students have connected with their bodies, I invite them to close their eyes and set a healing intention for the class.

I encourage my students to create an intention that is unique and meaningful to them.

It could be something specific to their yoga practice. Or it could also be related to something they are working through 'off the yoga mat'.

As the class unfolds, I remind them to bring their awareness back to their healing intention.

At the end of the session, I ask students to identify qualities they would like to take off the mat and into their life.

This approach helps me to create space for students to attune to what they want and need.

It also makes for a fun and interesting experience.

I have taught this body attunement and intention setting process for many years now. And can testify to the power of this healing tool.

Experiment with setting your own intention to *Heal Emotional Eating For Good*.

Healing intentions can be used in all areas of your life.

After my husband and I married, we decided to embark upon an exciting new adventure together.

We had spent the previous year living in Los Angeles and decided to return back to England to set up our lives.

We were looking for a renovation project we could pour all our love and energy into. The space also had to be one we could both live and work from.

We stumbled across an old Victorian property by the seaside. It was in a state of disrepair after years of neglect. Although the building appeared tired and unloved we could see it had potential. We thought we could transform the house by taking a healing approach to the renovations.

Before we embarked upon the renovations, my husband and I created a shared intention. We set our sights on co-creating a home that felt 'light and spacious'.

With our intention clarified, it was time to create our dream abode.

On the project we had many decisions to make everyday, both big and small. Each one had the ability to impact our end result. With each decision we asked ourselves, *"Will this help us to create a light and spacious home?"*

We worked with many different tradespeople on the project. This included architects, builders, carpenters, labourers, plumbers, electricians, plasterers, tilers and painters.

Each time we hired a new contractor, we shared our intention of creating a 'light and spacious' home. By sharing our intention our building team were better able to create the result we desired.

Like most renovations, our project ended up being bigger than we had anticipated. And we encountered many hurdles along the way. Our healing intention helped us to rise above our challenges and create a beautiful home that is a joy to live in.

Work with a healing guide

"What is a teacher? I'll tell you: it isn't someone who teaches something, but someone who inspires the student to give of her best in order to discover what she already knows."

~ Paulo Coelho

The morning after I made my choice to heal, I awoke exhausted.

I wanted to make a positive start to the rest of my life. So I dragged myself out of bed and prepared a healthy breakfast.

I was sitting at the kitchen table, adorned in my pyjamas, dressing gown and slippers. My old negative tape started running through my mind again.

After my euphoric decision to heal the previous night, doubts began entering my mind. It shook my confidence.

I found myself thinking things like; *"I feel terrible"*, *"Maybe I'm fooling myself?"* and *"What if my health doesn't improve and becomes even worse?"*

My mother entered the room, interrupting my thoughts. She took one look at me, placed her palm on my forehead.

"Missy you're running a fever" she said. *"You need to go straight back to bed"*.

When I woke later that morning, I found a small stack of books on my bed stand.

While I was sleeping, my mother had nipped down to our local library. She had borrowed some books on natural health and healing.

My parents lived in a small farming community. And I was amazed she was able to find reading material on the subject.

The selection of books lifted my spirits. I saw it as a confirmation that the Universe was starting to align with my healing intention.

My mother bought me a cup of fresh mint tea. I spent the afternoon propped up in my bed dipping in and out of the different titles.

It was an eye-opening experience. My initial review left me feeling waves of both excitement and overwhelm.

All the books seemed to confirm my intuition that it was possible to heal my body and my emotional eating. They recommended whole foods, natural medicine, gentle movement, cleansing protocols and relaxation techniques.

The books also made me feel a little anxious. This was all new to me. There seemed to be so much I didn't know and needed to learn.

I shared how I was feeling with my mother.

She told me there was no need for me to feel overwhelmed. All I needed to do was keep taking *"one small step at a time."*

My mother suggested we consult with a natural health practitioner. She thought they might be able to guide us through this new and unfamiliar landscape.

I felt a surge of relief wash over me at my mother's suggestion.

I knew I wanted to start my healing journey but was feeling so scared about having to go it alone.

I had struggled in the past because I had always felt uncomfortable reaching out for help. I didn't want people to perceive me as being weak or silly.

Breaking down was a humbling experience. It made me realise that seeking the right support was the very thing I needed to get well again.

I was grateful for the encouragement and support of my parents. Together, they became the bedrock of my healing team.

Finding my healing guide.

The following day, my mother contacted different healers, therapists and natural health practitioners.

She discussed my situation and scheduled a few appointments.

We met with each of them over the following weeks, as my energy and strength allowed.

They all had interesting things to share. But I didn't feel as if any of them could take me on the journey my soul was being guided to walk.

A friend then recommended I go and see her naturopath.

When I entered her healing practice, I immediately felt as if I had arrived home.

Her waiting room was warm and inviting. It contained a beautiful water feature, flowers and big green leafy plants.

The rippling sounds of water accompanied a subtle layer of background music. A delicate fragrance of lavender permeated the room.

Sitting in that tranquil environment, felt soothing for my body, mind and soul.

I felt my whole being-ness start to calm down and relax. It felt like the first time in forever.

The room appeared as if it were in a different realm to the clinical environment of my doctor's surgery.

The naturopath entered the room. She looked radiant and exuded an unmistakable aura of both softness and strength.

She introduced herself and then gave me a warm hug. She was unlike any woman I had ever encountered before.

I liked her immediately…

When we were sitting in her treatment room, she asked why I had come to see her?

I felt vulnerable yet so safe. I began to open up about my situation and my frustrations of being sick, tired and overweight.

It wasn't long before I started to weep. There was very little I could do to stop the tears so I surrendered to the moment.

For the first time since my body breakdown I allowed myself to experience my feelings. I felt tired and empty. I no longer had the strength to censor myself and my old emotions bubbled out of me.

Once I had regained my composure, the naturopath reached out and handed me a tissue.

"Your tears are a good thing..." she said. *"It's a sign your body is releasing all the tension it no longer needs to hold on to."*

The naturopath seemed so kind and accepting of my teary outburst. I didn't feel as if she was judging me or thinking I was a bad person.

Being in her presence and talking to her, made me feel like I was in a safe and protected space.

As I sat wiping the tears from my eyes, I became aware of how hard I had been working to hold everything together.

I hadn't realised how stressed and worn down I was.

I had been acting as if everything was 'okay' when clearly it wasn't.

She told me the reason why most women feel stressed is because they are trying to fit in and please other people.

"To heal and rebalance your body you need to start nourishing it..." she said. *"You also need to start being true to your self..."*

We had only just started working together and I already felt as if I had received a powerful healing...

"How do you work with your clients?" my mother asked.

"That's a great question..." she said. *"The simple answer is I work with my clients in a holistic way..."*

"We all have physical, mental and emotional aspects to our being. When any of these move out of balance it results in disharmony in our lives."

"Katrina's health challenges are symptoms of this imbalance. In order for her to heal her physical body, she will need to work upon her mental and emotional wellbeing as well..."

Our conversation made so much sense to me.

"Katrina, you may not realise this yet, but your sensitive and empathic nature is an amazing gift..." she said. *"One day you will use this gift to help guide and inspire others. But first we need to get you well again."*

I was a little lost for words.

No one had ever said anything like that to me before.

I had always seen my sensitive nature as a curse.

I felt as if I had been fully seen by another person for the first time in my life. I realised in that moment I had found my healing guide.

Over the next couple of years, my healing guide helped me to detoxify and nourish my physical body.

She also shared many different healing tools with me.

I used these tools to activate my intuition and regain my health and happiness.

These tools assisted me to rebalance my body, lose over 60 pounds and *Heal Emotional Eating For Good.*

Working with my healing guide also provided me with the inspiration to develop my own unique body of healing work.

Finding the right healing support.

Starting on the journey to heal the root causes of emotional eating can be a scary thing. For many women it involves stepping beyond what is comfortable and known.

The good news is you don't have to do it alone. Having a healing guide by your side can speed up your progress. It can also make the whole journey much more enjoyable.

Healing guides can be a great source of wisdom and inspiration. This is particularly true if they have completed their own healing journey.

A healing guide can help you navigate the twists and turns you will encounter along the path. They can also illuminate any blind spots you may have.

They can often see you in a way that your friends and family don't. And can also help you to release the past and encourage you to start moving in the direction of your dreams.

Now although I was fortunate enough to have my own personal healing guide, it is not always necessary. There are many different support options available for women today. Particularly when you consider the wealth of information available on the internet.

Support can come in many different forms. This can include inspirational articles and blogs or reading books like this one.

You might also like to attend yoga classes, meditation workshops and healing retreats. There are many great audio recordings and home study programs available as well.

Choose support that works for you on your healing journey. Be mindful of your unique circumstances and trust your intuition.

Remember this is your life. You can choose to surround yourself with people who can help you to become all you can be.

* To help you get started I have created a FREE meditation recording. Download it now from www.HealEmotionalEating.net.

Chapter summary.

Phase 2 of the healing journey starts the moment you choose to heal.

Before making the choice to heal you may hear yourself saying something like *"I can't go on like this any longer"*. Or even *"there has to be more to life than this..."*

When you choose to heal, you become willing and open to change.

And also ready to do something different.

It can be a very powerful and life-defining moment.

Once you have chosen to heal the next step is to set your healing intention.

Visualise your healing intention manifesting with ease and grace.

Use it to ground your dreams into reality and create healthy routines and habits that work for you.

As you progress along your healing journey, choose to work alongside a healing guide.

Work with someone who has already created the results you want to achieve. Also ensure the guide is someone you resonate with.

Be kind and patient with yourself as you make your way along your healing journey.

It takes time to release the past and grow into the person you are capable of becoming.

Trust in the healing process and enjoy each step of the way.

Chapter Six – Clear Your Clutter

"Sometimes you've got to let everything go - purge yourself. If you are unhappy with anything... whatever is bringing you down, get rid of it. Because you'll find that when you're free, your true creativity, your true self comes out..."

~ Tina Turner

Become conscious of your clutter

"The ability to simplify means to eliminate the unnecessary so that the necessary may speak."

~ Hans Hofmann

Natasha booked a *Breakthrough Healing Session* to find a way to deal with her stress and emotional eating.

She held a managerial role and would regularly work long hours.

Natasha said her staple diet consisted of *"coffee, carbs and cigarettes"*.

She shared she had a *"gnawing feeling in the pit of her gut"*. And it would only go away after she ate bread, pasta or hot chips.

Working on Natasha's emotional eating at that point would have only added to her stress levels.

We instead started to look for alternative ways to reduce her stress load.

I asked Natasha about her personal life outside of work. I was curious to find out how she managed everything given her rigorous schedule.

She admitted her job made it difficult to stay connected with members of her family.

She said it also made it hard to maintain friendships outside of work. Or consider the possibility of romance.

"How do you manage everything at home?" I asked.

Natasha started sobbing.

I offered her a tissue and gave her the space to be with her emotions.

"My spare bedroom is so full of stuff it's overwhelming..." Natasha confessed. *"I can barely open the door anymore..."*

I asked Natasha to tell me more…

Natasha said she used the room to store the belongings she had inherited from her mother.

Natasha revealed she still hadn't dealt with the grief from her mother's death. Even though she had passed a few years earlier.

The spare room had morphed into a physical manifestation of her emotional world.

"I wouldn't know where to start…" she said. *"And I don't have the time or emotional energy to sort through it all on my own."*

With Natasha's permission we began to do some emotional release work to clear the stuck energy. Natasha was being very brave and I soon felt her heavy emotions start to shift.

By the end of the session she was filled with gratitude for her mothers life. She also committed to starting a new chapter for herself.

"What would you like to use the bedroom for instead?" I asked.

She shared with me she had always dreamed of starting her own business. She thought the room would make the perfect *"home office"*.

We then brainstormed different people she could ask to support her through the clearing process.

When I spoke to Natasha a few weeks later she told me an old family friend had helped her to clear the room.

She said they had a *"fun weekend together"*. They sorted through her mother's things and shared stories about her life. She placed all the sentimental items to one side and then gifted everything else to charity.

She told me she had bought herself a new desk. And was transforming her spare bedroom into her dream home office.

She added she was feeling more optimistic and in control of her life. And the *'gnawing feeling in her gut'* had disappeared…

The link between clutter and stress.

As we move through the healing protocol, we will focus on ways to reduce stress at the root of emotional eating.

One of the most effective ways to reduce environmental stress is to clear clutter from your life.

Or in other words discard objects that don't serve a practical function or bring you enjoyment.

Clearing clutter is a great healing tool for relieving residual stress and anxiety.

Reducing my clutter over the years has helped me to release the things I had outgrown. And also create more space for the things I value.

I first learnt about clearing clutter when I was in my mid 20s.

I was browsing the self-development section of my favourite bookstore.

As I pulled a book from the shelf, I knocked another to the ground.

I reached down and picked up the book with the intention of returning it back to the slot from which it fell.

As I did, the books elegant cover and typeface caught my eye.

The book was on clearing clutter. I was intrigued. So I sat myself down cross-legged on the floor and started to dip into its pages.

The book shared many incredible insights.

Including how our physical environments are a reflection of our internal ones.

The book had me enthralled.

I felt so inspired to start clearing my own clutter I jumped up, walked over to the cashier and bought the book.

Becoming conscious of my clutter.

When I arrived home I decided to walk around and notice where my clutter 'lived'. I was curious about which area I would feel inspired to clear first.

I was sharing a modest one-bedroom apartment with my then boyfriend. So it was pretty easy for me to be able to whiz around.

I started my clutter assessment in the kitchen. I opened cupboards, looked inside drawers and observed bench space.

It was fascinating to look at the space energetically for the first time.

Everywhere I looked seemed to be busy and overflowing with 'things'. And this was despite our joint efforts to keep things 'clean'.

I then moved into the lounge room and dining area to carry on the process. I was surprised by how much stuff we had accumulated between us and wondered what it all represented.

It became obvious our home lacked a systematic way to organise our possessions.

My next step was to assess the bedroom. I scanned the room. On the surface it appeared to be tidy and in good order.

That was until I swung open the doors of our shared wardrobe.

I took a moment to observe the space. The wardrobe was a decent size. It was inbuilt and divided in two.

We had arranged the space in a 'his and her' style setup. I noticed my boyfriends' side was much tidier than mine and felt a twinge of shame.

My clothes rail was packed tight with dresses, jackets and coats. I had stuff popping out everywhere.

I looked at the clothes hanging in my wardrobe and realised there were many things I rarely wore.

I had a set of drawers inside the wardrobe where I stored my clothing items such as my t-shirts, socks and lingerie.

Each drawer I opened was overflowing and in a state of chaos.

I then looked down at the floor of the wardrobe. It was covered with an assortment of my shoes, bags and belts.

The final part of my wardrobe assessment was the top shelf that sat above everything. I used this area to store all my paper work. It was in disarray. Filled with notebooks, journals, folders, bills, letters, books, birthday cards and bank statements.

It became obvious my wardrobe was the place I needed to clear first. I felt a strong urge to take action and get everything sorted before my boyfriend returned home.

I began the clutter clearing process by removing all the items from my side of the wardrobe.

I organised everything into two separate piles on the floor.

Pile 1: Things to discard.
Pile 2: Things to keep.

Once I had removed every item from my wardrobe, I then vacuumed the inside and wiped the shelves clean.

I took a moment to appreciate how great the empty storage looked. I was determined to maintain the simplicity of the space by only returning the items I used and loved.

In my 'discard' pile were items that belonged in my past. This included clothes I hadn't worn in the last 12 months.

I added to this pile any clothes that didn't fit me as well as items in a poor state of repair. I then bagged up the stuff to either take to the charity shop or to drop into the trash.

In my 'keep' pile were all the items I wanted to take forward into my future. It included the clothes I still used and loved.

After I had returned these items back to the wardrobe, I took a moment to admire them.

I was delighted with the end result and exhaled a big sigh of relief.

The wardrobe looked incredible.

It felt far more organised and functional. Each item of clothing now had allocated space and a place to call 'home'.

It looked so good. I wondered if it would inspire my boyfriend to release and let go of some of his old clothes!

I had almost finished sorting everything. And then I came across my small collection of treasured books lying on the ground.

These books were on healing, spirituality and self-development. I had collected the different titles over many years.

I had pushed these books to the back of my wardrobe when we moved into the flat. I had forgotten all about them.

Seeing my books once again was like reconnecting with dear friends.

As I thumbed through the pages, I yearned to re-read them.

It didn't feel right to throw them out or for me to give them away.

And I no longer could bear the thought of having them hidden away in my wardrobe either.

My special books deserved a proper home.

I wanted to have them on display in the living room so I could dip in and out of them whenever I wanted to.

I wiped the cover of each book and placed them into a cardboard box. I then carried them into the living room.

The bookshelf in the living room was filled to the brim. It became obvious what my next clutter clearing project was going to be...

Becoming conscious of your clutter.

If you are like most people, you are much better at acquiring things than you are at releasing them.

This natural tendency results in the gradual accumulation of 'stuff' over time. It can also create feelings of chaos, disorganisation and being 'out of control.'

If this pattern remains unaddressed, our lives can soon become overloaded with things. This can make life feel heavy, burdensome and difficult to manage.

We can end up restricting our spirits with all the stuff we have collected along the way. So much so, it can inhibit the ability to enjoy the present moment or get excited about the future.

Our homes can morph into shrines of the past. Rather than be open and flowing spaces filled with future possibility.

To turn this tide around, it's important to pay attention to the possessions you have gathered.

Many women ask me, *'Katrina, I would love to clear my clutter... I've been meaning to do it for ages. But, I'm not sure how to get started?'*

Maybe you are feeling the same way?

I have found the best way to begin the process is to start 'becoming conscious of your clutter'. Yes, that's right - you can get started, without lifting a finger.

Becoming conscious of your clutter involves taking a closer look at your things.

The goal at this stage is to build an awareness of your clutter and where it lives. And you can do this without taking any action to sort it out.

This will help you to understand your patterns and habits around clutter. As you gain awareness this will assist you to release it, as well as prevent it from building up again in the future.

Becoming 'clutter conscious' means to notice the things that annoy and frustrate you. It also involves identifying areas you feel inspired and motivated to get sorted out.

Pay special attention to the things you already know you are ready to release. Doing this will help you to quickly build momentum as you start clearing clutter later on.

As you become conscious of your clutter notice which items do not have a 'home', as well as those that do.

I like to give each of my possessions a home. After I use them, it is nice to return them back to where they belong.

If things are not given a home it can create feelings of overwhelm. This can trigger coping strategies such as emotional eating.

Once you have become conscious of your clutter you will be ready to start your first project.

You can start with any area you feel inspired to get sorted out. I started clearing clutter in my wardrobe.

Clearing your clutter will help you to complete on the past. It will also reduce the amount of environmental stress you are exposed to.

This will help you to feel lighter, more organised and in control of your life. It will also reduce your desire for emotional eating.

As you put things in their right place, real healing can occur.

With practice, your clutter clearing abilities will grow and develop. With each area you clear you will gain more energy and momentum. This will give you the necessary strength and skill to tackle bigger projects in the future.

I have created an exercise on the following few pages called *'Assess Your Clutter'*.

This will help you to start becoming aware of your clutter and identify the areas to work on first.

Exercise: Assess your clutter.

Fill out the assessment forms below to start building awareness of your clutter.

a) Physical clutter assessment form.

Physical clutter assessment form.	Over capacity (Yes / No)	Inspired to declutter? (Yes / No)
Purse		
Handbag		
Shoe rack		
Wardrobe		
Bedroom 1		
Bedroom 2		
Bedroom 3		
Kitchen cupboards		
Refrigerator		
Home office		
Desk		
Bookshelf		
Car		
Garage		
Attic / basement		

b) Paper clutter assessment form.

Paper clutter assessment form.	Over capacity? (Yes / No)	Inspired to declutter? (Yes / No)
Regular mail		
Junk mail and circulars		
Magazines		
Household bills		
Bank statements		
Folders		
Storage shelves		
Filing cabinets		
Journals and diaries		
Scrap books		
Photo albums		
Birthday cards		
Sentimental letters		
Course notes		
Creative projects		
Certificates		
Tax returns		
Any other paper clutter		

c) Digital clutter assessment form.

Digital clutter assessment form.	Over capacity? (Yes / No)	Inspired to declutter? (Yes / No)
Email inbox		
Computer files		
Computer desktop icons		
Digital photos		
Digital videos		
Email newsletters		
Social media profiles		
Online passwords		
Online banking		
Online bill payments		
Online subscriptions		
Direct debits		
Phone apps		
Digital backups		
Digital storage and usb sticks		
Old cell phones and cameras		
Old cables, cords and remotes		
Software manuals		

Clear clutter in your kitchen

"Happiness is a place between too little and too much."

~ Finnish Proverb

Patricia was a self-employed designer. She had a vivacious spirit that lit up any room she walked into.

She booked a series of *Breakthrough Healing Sessions* with me to work on her emotional eating.

"I am someone who has struggled with weight problems my entire life" Patricia said. *"I have done many things to try and change my situation but I still feel as if I am blocked and holding on. I love your kind and gentle approach and was wondering if you could help me?"*

Managing both her clients and cash flow were big sources of ongoing stress and worry for her.

She often found herself working *"crazy hours or not at all"*.

She found both scenarios stressful and said they had a negative impact upon her state of being.

"Katrina, I'm in great resistance and self harm mode at the moment. I've lost faith that anything will ever work for me after years of internal battle and struggle."

I asked Patricia how she dealt with her stress levels?

"The thing that helps me feel better is food" she said. *"Especially heavy foods like cheese, breads, pasta and ice cream. I'm not much of a cook and I like to eat out... Wine and vodka seem to do the trick too."*

"I'm concerned I have left it too late" she said. *"I worry nothing will ever work for me... And it's in this scared state I crave comfort and make poor food choices."*

I suggested to Patricia we do a **Kitchen Decluttering Session**.

I wanted to see if we could reduce the stress she was experiencing at home and set her up for success.

After a warm welcome at Patricia's home, I asked if she would like to give me a tour of her kitchen. I suggested she take her time and point out anything that stood out for her.

Patricia started the tour by introducing me to her kitchen cupboards.

The first thing she noticed were all the different food items crammed into the space. She said she had purchased many of the items on her overseas travels.

"Katrina I love to travel and I always bring back specialty food items from my trips. The trouble is, I very rarely use the ingredients to prepare meals with when I get home. And they end up cluttering my valuable cupboard space..."

"That's a great distinction" I replied. *"What else do you notice?"*

The next thing Patricia pointed out was a dinnerware set at the top of her cupboard.

"I do love these plates but I can't remember the last time I used them... I'm someone who craves human connection almost as much as food... I bought the set for special occasions but because they are hard for me to reach I don't often pull them down..."

We carried on with the kitchen tour until we arrived at the final destination - the refrigerator.

"When I buy fresh fruits and vegetables, I often find myself throwing them out" she said. *"Due to my unpredictable schedule they generally go off before I have a chance to prepare them..."*

I could relate to all the things Patricia was sharing.

I thanked her for the tour. I enjoyed both the stories and insights she shared with me as we made our way around her kitchen.

The kitchen is the heart of a home.

Some of my earliest memories were in the kitchen and I've always felt this special room to be the heart of the home.

I was active in the kitchen from a young age and had a real passion for baking. My specialty items were cakes, cookies and slices.

I lost my connection with the kitchen when I left home to attend boarding school.

As all my meals were prepared for me, I had little need to put my cooking skills to use.

When my body broke down I contemplated the role kitchens play in creating health.

My healing guide said if I wanted to lose weight, it was essential I set my kitchen up right. She said an organised kitchen was foundational in creating health.

With her encouragement I transformed my kitchen into my *'Healing Headquarters'*.

This gave me the opportunity to rediscover my passion for cooking. Only this time, I was able to do so in a much healthier way.

"Katrina, it's our private eating habits that tend to sabotage our success… Rather than what we allow ourselves to eat in public" my healing guide said. *"That is why it's essential you pay attention to the foods you eat when no one else is watching."*

Due to this she encouraged me to remove any fake foods from my kitchen that could cause my body harm.

She said it would be a good idea to replace them with whole foods and natural ingredients. This was so I could prepare healthy snacks as well as quick and easy meals whenever I was hungry.

This one insight shifted my awareness and helped me to transform my eating habits.

Discarding excess.

Once Patricia had taken stock of her kitchen, it was time to start clearing clutter.

I shared the aim of clearing clutter was to remove unused and unloved objects from the home.

The reason we do this is to have more space for the things that are important and useful in our lives.

It would also help her to feel happy, balanced and peaceful in the kitchen. Which would lead her to making better food choices.

When it comes to clearing clutter it is always a good idea to work on one area at a time. This helps to avoid overwhelm.

I asked Patricia where she wanted to start.

"The cupboards!" she replied.

We began clearing everything out of her cupboards and placing them on her kitchen bench. We then rolled up our sleeves and wiped down the shelves until they sparkled and shined.

Our next task was to work out which items would go back on the shelves and which we would discard.

To simplify this task we began grouping items together in piles.

She identified the food items she wanted to keep.

We then discarded anything that was either out of date, duplicates or ones she knew she would never use.

"Spices Katrina" Patricia laughed. *"I have enough here to last me lifetimes!"*

We used the same approach with her fridge. We ended up discarding old food and an assortment of half-empty condiment jars and bottles.

Our next project was to sort through her crockery, cups and glassware. Once again, we grouped similar items together to make it easier to sort.

I asked her to discard any unloved, unused, broken or chipped items.

"Patricia, what's the perfect number of plates, bowls, cups, and glasses for your needs?"

"I occasionally have friends or family over for dinner" she said. *"So I guess eight of each should be enough..."*

I encouraged her to select her favourite items and place them in an easy to access area of her cupboard.

"Using your special plates and glasses on a daily basis is a great reminder that each meal is a sacred act..." I said.

We placed surplus items into boxes to drop off at a charity shop. We had also collected a garbage bag of old food items and clutter to go into the trash.

Once we had returned the essential items back to the cupboards, Patricia and I stood back to admire them.

Everything was visible and much easier to access. There was also room to spare on the shelves, which had a calming effect.

"I feel so much lighter already!" Patricia said. *"It makes me want to get to work on the other areas of my house too!"*

In our next session Patricia shared she had experienced a real breakthrough.

She said she felt calmer and more connected to her body.

"Katrina, with food, I am so much better. When I go to the fridge, I now check in with my body and ask it what it wants to eat. The other day, I got the answer – melon. So I cut up some cubes of melon..."

"And then my mind wanted coffee... but when I asked my body, it said it wanted water... So I had a glass of water with a slice of lemon..."

Clearing clutter leads to healing.

Clearing clutter is an effective way to heal incomplete emotional experiences.

This is why I recommend clearing clutter as a great place to start your own process of emotional healing.

Clutter can serve as a visual cue to what is going on in your inner world. It can also provide profound insights as to the nature of your emotional eating.

Your clutter is a mirror of your inner world. It can provide you with clues as to what remains neglected and unfinished in your life.

It can also reveal mental and emotional blocks you may have. Including limiting beliefs that keep you feeling stuck.

Clearing clutter is a great way to release accumulated stress and stagnant energy.

It gives you the chance to let go of the burdens of your past.

When you clear clutter, you get to see the connection you have with your possessions.

As you release your clutter you will lighten your stress load.

With awareness you can let go of the things that no longer serve you. This includes your physical possessions, as well as old mental and emotional patterns.

Clearing clutter enables you to process the past in a positive way and complete upon it.

This creates more space for the person you are growing into rather than holding on to the person you once were.

Know that with each unwanted item you release, you are healing another little part of you.

From mess and stress to success.

When you clear clutter, you are not only cleaning up your external environment, but your inner one too.

As you release the things you no longer need, you release emotional attachments to your past.

It is important to be aware that this process of clearing clutter can bring up strong emotions.

If you feel emotional at any stage, grant yourself the space to be with your feelings.

The key is to express and release any old emotional entanglements as well.

Be aware of this and use gentle healing tools to support you through this process.

Affirmations are a great healing tool to use as you clear your clutter.

One of my favourite healing affirmations is…

"It's safe to let go."

As you release stress and excess, you create new future possibilities for your life. It will also help you to create space for what matters.

If you have a lot of clutter, take your time. Select one area and break the job into small and manageable baby steps.

This is especially important if you experience any feelings of overwhelm.

It's also worth remembering you don't have to do it alone. Do you have a friend or family member who could help you?

You could also hire a clutter clearing professional to support you with this process.

Exercise: Clutter clearing project.

Here is a practical set of steps to assist you with your next clutter clearing project.

Tip #1 - Select your project: Use the *Clutter Assessment Form* to select your next clutter clearing project.

Look for the area you feel most inspired to get sorted out and start there.

Tip #2 – Your keep pile: As you clear your space, connect with your possessions. Notice how they feel. You can ask yourself:

"Does this item belong to my past or is it part of my future?"

If the item is part of your future, keep it and give it a home. Also be sure the item is one you either love or use regularly.

If you feel uncertain about whether to discard an item ask yourself, *"Would I purchase this item today?"*

And if the answer is yes, then ask yourself, *"How much would I be prepared to pay for it?"*

Tip #3 – Your discard pile: Give yourself a time limit to discard your unwanted items. This is particularly important for items you wish to sell, donate or give away.

Keep in mind the key to successful clutter clearing is to move unwanted items on swiftly.

Tip #4 – After you have cleared the space: Take the clutter you wish to discard out of your house as soon as you can.

Drop unwanted items into a charity shop, recycling depot or garbage bin.

Once you have cleared your clutter, it is time to turn your attention to creating sacred space in your life...

Create sacred space

"Your sacred space is where you can find yourself over and over again."

~ Joseph Campbell

My box of books sat on the living room floor for the next couple of weeks. I wanted to give them the home they deserved but I didn't know how to go about it.

Our living room bookshelf was filled with my boyfriend's books, folders and magazines.

I'm sure he would have been happy to clear some space for me if I had asked him to.

The problem was I didn't want to.

It was an awkward feeling to have to sit with. It wasn't so much about my boyfriend, the bookshelf or even the books themselves.

What I was most concerned about was what the books said about me.

I had never felt safe enough to reveal my interest in personal growth and spirituality. Not even with my boyfriend.

I had always been afraid if other people saw my books they might judge or criticise me. Or worse, they would think I was 'some kind of weirdo' and not want to be my friend anymore.

This was why I had stored my books at the back of my closet in the first place when I moved into the flat.

My second clutter clearing project had brought up a confronting question…

Did I have the courage to reveal, honour and cherish the things that were important to me?

An act of self-love.

It dawned on me I couldn't expect others to love and accept me, if I wasn't prepared to love and accept myself first.

Hiding my true self wasn't an act of love. Nor was hiding away my favourite books in my closet.

I realised it wasn't enough to love the 'self' I thought other people wanted to see. What I needed to do was love the 'me' that was a whole and authentic expression of my true self.

I could see I had a real opportunity to transform my predicament. Rather than ask my boyfriend to give up space on our existing bookshelf, I decided to create my own.

I pledged my new bookshelf would be a symbolic gesture of my desire to be true to myself. I wanted a way to honour all the different parts of me I had kept hidden for so long.

I mustered the nerve to drive down to my local hardware store.

A grandfatherly shop assistant must have sensed my apprehension. He asked me if I needed help.

I shared I wanted to create a new bookshelf. I confided with him I had never attempted a 'DIY project' before. I was unsure of where to start and questioned my ability to complete such a task.

He assured me building a bookshelf was not as hard as it seemed.

He said the store sold special shelf building kits. He said they contained everything I would need to get the job done. Including step-by-step instructions.

He then walked me down to the appropriate aisle.

After I paid for the shelf kit, I thanked the assistant for his help. He had given me the confidence I needed to give the project a go.

I then went home to build my shelves…

Creating sacred space.

Clearing clutter is an important part of healing your emotional eating. It isn't however the final destination to reduce stress in your physical environment.

The ultimate goal is to create an environment where you feel safe to be yourself. This is what I like to call 'sacred space'.

Sacred space allows a woman to feel comfortable, relaxed and at home within her own skin.

When you feel safe to be yourself, you will make better food choices. You will naturally want to consume foods that are healing for your body and avoid foods that aren't.

When you feel safe you will be more able to prioritise your self-care. This includes dedicating time and resources towards things that support your healing journey.

The opposite of sacred space is 'unsafe space'.

An **unsafe space** is an environment where you do not feel safe to be yourself. When you don't feel safe, it is only natural to feel a desire for protection. This can trigger bouts of emotional eating.

Unsafe spaces make you feel fearful, judged, criticised, threatened, defensive or vulnerable. In unsafe spaces women feel the need to comfort or defend themselves.

Some of my clients have shared they do not feel safe in their jobs and workplaces.

This can be particularly harmful given the amount of time they spend there each week.

Others say they feel overwhelmed in supermarkets, shopping malls or other public spaces.

We often can't influence the nature of public spaces. This is why it is essential we create sacred space in our personal environments.

Creating sacred space at home.

When my boyfriend came home from work, he noticed the bookshelf.

"Hey, who gave you the new book shelf?" he asked.

"Oh, I built it myself" I replied.

"Yeah right!" he laughed.

"Seriously, who gave you the bookshelf?"

"I told you, I built it myself."

When he saw that I wasn't laughing, he walked over to inspect the bookshelf.

"You built this? How?"

"Well I went down to the hardware store... and I met this lovely shop assistant... and he assured me I could do it..."

"Okay, but why did you build this?"

I took a deep breath. I then opened up about how I'd been feeling about my books.

"I wanted my books to have a home. They are important to me and I felt upset I didn't have a special place for them..."

He re-examined the shelf.

"Well your books look happy in their new home. I'm impressed with your handy work... You've done a good job and you should feel proud of yourself."

My eyes misted over and I felt my heart expand.

He then walked over to me and gave me a hug...

Chapter summary.

Clearing clutter is an act of loving kindness to your self.

It reduces environmental stress, creates balance and a feeling of flow.

In the beginning this healing process is likely to feel unfamiliar. It may even feel a little uncomfortable. Keep going anyway.

Releasing excess is an essential part of the healing journey.

As you clear your physical clutter, you release the past and heal old wounds. You will feel more powerful, focused and organised. It will also reduce your desire for emotional eating.

With less clutter, you create space for what is important. This will also help you to access deeper levels of your intuition.

Once you have cleared your clutter you can turn your attention to creating sacred space in your life.

Sacred space is where you feel safe to be yourself. It is also a place for deep rest, renewal and rejuvenation.

The more you connect to sacred space, the stronger the bond to your true self will become.

You can start to create sacred space in your life with a very small act. You can arrange flowers, frame a photo or even roll out your yoga mat.

Connecting to your sacred space on a regular basis is the key to creating authentic success. Allow this process to give you the confidence and courage to connect with your true feelings.

As you grow and feel safe to express more of who you are, your sacred space will expand too.

With time, your sacred space will extend into every aspect of your life.

Chapter Seven – Care For Your Body

"Unlike much of orthodox medicine, alternative approaches to healing typically honour the wisdom and capability of the human body. Their goal is often to support and strengthen the powerful healing forces already at work within us."

~ John Robbins

Listen to your body

"The body is a sacred garment: it is what you enter life in and what you depart life with, and it should be treated with honour and with joy..."

~ Martha Graham

Here's a sweet email I received from Cherrie a reader of my first book *Losing Weight is a Healing Journey*.

***

Dear Katrina,

I'm a nurse working on a busy ER floor in a hospital.

A few months ago at work I had a complete breakdown. It was due to all the feelings of stress I was experiencing in my life.

After collapsing at work I took a good look at myself. Lots of tears and prayers later, I decided enough was enough.

During that time I came across an article you wrote online. It was about losing weight by going on a healing journey.

It caught my eye not only because I have some weight to lose but because you called it a 'healing journey'.

Everything you said made so much sense to me... I felt it was the right time to start taking better care of myself.

I wanted to heal my body, regain my energy and feel joyful once again. I read many articles on your website, ordered your book and bought your Yoga DVD program.

I'm starting to feel so much better. I am more positive and joyful. I love life and I no longer cry all the time.

I've been fighting for years to get my energy back and to discover who I am.

Sometimes, when it's quiet at home, I ask my body how it feels... And it's amazing what I'm discovering!

My body has taught me it doesn't like dairy... so I have stopped eating it. I'm taking baby steps to reduce sugar and gluten too.

I've decreased my pasta intake to once a week and I'm happy with that... It's incredible because I'm a cheese and pasta lover!

I am going to give myself about a year to get back into shape. I'm learning how to listen to my body and take care of it for the first time.

I eat healthy foods and lots of veggies because I love them, not because I have to.

I no longer use food to escape my emotions. I express them now instead. When I'm sad, I cry. When I'm tired, I sleep. When I'm bored, I create something.

I have a reminder in my little sewing studio that says: "This is my healing journey. I nourish my body, my mind, my emotions and my soul joyfully".

It's going to be a long and bumpy journey, but it's so exciting... I'm starting to love this body that I have with all its imperfections.

I used to use food as a comforter, but not anymore, because I am learning how to listen to and love my body.

I'm not yet done with all my goals, but I have lost weight, regained my energy and I have my joy back!

And I know that healing is a journey and I love it.

Love Cherrie

***

A culture of override.

When I receive emails from readers like Cherrie I feel heartened.

It fills me with joy to hear stories of women re-discovering this sacred connection with themselves.

Something magical happens when a woman listens to her body.   I know this re-orientation offers many gifts.

It opens the door for her to not only feel healthier but to also start living a life she loves.

By listening to her body, she is able to move beyond the conditioning and expectations of society. It also gives her access to greater levels of her intuition.

This act helps build the courage to be true to her self and create authentic success and genuine happiness.

 It will also give her the space to be present for what's most important.

Today we live in a culture that encourages women to override their bodies.   The pressure and expectations placed on women to be successful has never been higher.

When you override your body with emotional eating, you are silencing its intelligence.

Overriding your body through force means to push it beyond its natural capacity. If this continues for long enough it can move your body out of balance. It can even lead to physical breakdown.

I learnt this lesson the hard way. I used to override my body by suppressing my true needs and desires with fake food.

In the beginning, my body would send me gentle messages to express it wasn't happy. Of course I didn't listen to them and the knocks became louder.

Even then, I continued to ignore them…

My body fired a warning shot.

An outside voice penetrated my absent mind, *"Is everything okay?"*

A waitress stood across from my table with a concerned look on her face.

I must have been staring at my coffee a little longer than was normal.

It was a Sunday morning and I was sitting in the cafe across the road from my work. I had a part time university job at a shoe store and my shift was about to start in less than 20 minutes.

I cleared my throat and assured her that I was fine.

I'm not sure I was particularly convincing, but she smiled and went back to clearing tables.

The truth was I didn't feel fine. Far from it.

I felt like I was nursing a hangover. The only trouble being, I hadn't been drinking.

If I was completely honest with myself, I hadn't felt right for a while.

My sleep patterns were out and my adrenals were shot.

In the evenings I would feel wired and unable to sleep. And then in the mornings my alarm clock would struggle to rouse me.

I'd also been gaining weight.

It seemed as if I only had to give food a sideways glance and I would be wearing it the next day.

I reached over to grab the cup with my right hand.

It was shaking.

I dropped my hand back under the table before anyone noticed...

Something seemed wrong with my body.

My heart raced and my throat tightened.

My breath became all short and heavy. It reminded me of some of the unforgiving asthma attacks I suffered as a child.

I knew I had to somehow pull myself together. Fast.

I squeezed my left palm with my right hand in an attempt to settle my nerves.

Calling in sick was not an option.

If I did, I knew that I would be putting my job on the line.

The store employed university students to work the weekend shifts. And my boss was well aware of our carefree attitudes.

She had cautioned us about *"pulling sickies"*, particularly on Sunday mornings.

And besides, my rent was due and I needed the money.

My mind intervened in an attempt to raise my sluggish bones.

"Come on Katrina, get yourself together... Stop being so dramatic... You're over-reacting..."

I dug deep and lifted the cup to my lips.

It was a strong brew and it seemed to give my body the jolt it needed.

I wasn't drinking the coffee for pleasure. I was drinking it to try and kick-start my weary body.

After I emptied the cup, I asked the waitress if she could put my chocolate chip muffin in a takeaway bag.

I then stood up and crossed the road to work...

Overriding your body with fake food.

When you override your body with fake food you create 'fake energy'. When you do this, you start to live on an energy source that is not your own.

Fake energy can come from coffee, sugar, soda, fake food, alcohol and even certain drugs.

These substances can give you an instant kick or energy boost.

These spikes in energy are temporary. Energy crashes can follow leaving you feeling much worse.

Consuming fake food increases the stress on your body. It can affect your hormones, pancreas, liver and digestive system.

These fake sources of energy can be addictive.

The more you consume, the more your body will need to function. This dynamic sets up a destructive cravings cycle that can be difficult to break out of.

With time your body will come to rely more and more on these fake sources of energy.

Fake foods can interfere with your sleep, moods and general feelings of wellbeing. The longer you use these fake sources of energy, the more detrimental effects they will have.

Before my body breakdown, coffee and sugar were my 'drugs of choice'. They provided my body with the fake energy I craved to get me through the day.

The more I consumed these fake sources of energy the more depleted my body became.

This in turn intensified my cravings for instant hits of fake energy.

Fake foods led me to feeling tired and on the verge of total exhaustion.

Breaking the spell of fake energy.

To *Heal Emotional Eating For Good* switch your body's fuel source from 'fake energy' to 'real energy'.

Real energy comes from living in harmony with your unique truth. This involves respecting your body's natural rhythm and intelligence.

Real energy comes from drinking clean water and eating real foods. It also comes from moving your body, spending time in nature and keeping good sleep patterns.

Women get themselves into trouble when they override their bodies with their minds. This is often done to keep up with the expectations they place upon themselves as well as those of others.

To break this dynamic, place your body's needs above the desire for social approval.

I know this can be particularly challenging for women. We have a natural tendency to place the needs of others above our own.

On my healing journey I had to learn how to 'fill my own well' first. I discovered my inner 'no'.

Instead of giving my energy, love and attention to others, I began to prioritise my needs above all else. Re-orientating myself in this way helped me to transform my life.

By saying 'no' to others, it meant I could start saying 'yes' to myself. Once I had recovered my health and happiness, I was then able to give to others from a more authentic place.

It is important you create the space for your body to speak. It has its own language that often gets drowned out by the chatter of the mind.

One of my favourite healing tools is to find the hidden gift in pain. Rather than supress it with food, ask what new insights your pain is trying to bring you.

What I discovered for myself is that awareness is curative.

Exercise: Building body awareness.

Use the following exercise to give you clues as to where you are currently overriding your body.

Tick the sentences you feel apply to you…

Are you overriding your body?	Yes / No
I need coffee and/or sugar to get through my day.	
I eat fake food when I feel bored, upset or lonely.	
I use fake food to give me energy boosts.	
I frequently eat fake food when I am alone.	
I frequently over eat and then feel uncomfortable.	
I find it hard to stop eating, even when I want to.	
I overeat and drink in social settings.	
I drink soda (and/or diet drinks) on a regular basis.	
I drink alcohol at night to take the edge off my day.	
I experience aches, pain and discomfort in my body.	
I feel disconnected from my body's true needs.	
I wake up in the morning feeling tired and exhausted.	
I feel alert in the evenings, especially around bedtime.	
I habitually override my body.	
I force myself to exercise even though I don't enjoy it.	
I feel overburdened by social obligations.	

Awaken your body

"There is deep wisdom within our very flesh, if we can only come to our senses and feel it."

~ Elizabeth A. Behnke

Georgie booked a coaching session to work on her emotional eating. She also wanted to rediscover her *"joie de vivre"*.

She was an artist living and working in London.

We decided to meet in one of my favourite health food cafés in the city.

We sat down at a large wooden table and we both ordered a green juice.

"Katrina, when my relationship broke down, my whole life fell apart."

Georgie shared she had separated from her husband and was starting her life anew.

"I wasn't expecting to have to start over at this stage of my life... I fell into a dark abyss... I had nowhere to live... I had all these financial worries... and I felt like I couldn't turn to any of our shared friends...

I asked her how she managed to cope with such challenging circumstances...

"It is fair to say I didn't cope very well. I threw myself into my work. I work on my own so this was quite lonely... I started eating take away food... I drank too much red wine and binged on chocolate..."

I then asked Georgie what her intention was for our session?

"Well I've finally come to a place within myself where I feel ready to make a fresh start."

"I know I need to take better care of my body. I am also hopeful this might give me the courage and confidence to start dating again..."

I said, *"That sounds great and..."*

Georgie leant across the table. *"Katrina, do you really think I can heal my emotional eating? Or have I left it too late?"*

"I feel so frumpy..." she said. *"My belly feels swollen. My arms wobble and my thighs jiggle... I hate feeling like this..."*

"I can feel myself getting older. My body feels tired and stiff. Plus, I have these dark circles gathering under my eyes. And, to top it off, I have all these grey hairs wiggling through..."

"These days I have to drag myself out of bed and force myself to face the day. I don't know if I can stop myself from eating all the foods I know are so bad for me... I feel like my body has let me down... But, I also know I haven't been treating it right either."

"Georgie, I can relate to how you feel" I said. *"I used to believe it would be impossible for me to change. That was until my healing guide said it was possible for me to transform my life..."*

"Once I believed that change could happen everything started to shift. A whole new world opened up to me. I started learning all about my body and focused upon improving my daily habits..."

"I began to see my body as my friend and not my enemy. With this new approach my body started to respond..."

"Do you think I can do this too?" Georgie asked.

I reached across the table and held Georgie's hand.

"Of course I think you can... But what is more important than what I think, is what you think. If you believe you can... you will."

We had a great session together with lots of laughs and ah-ha moments.

To help her on her journey, I emailed Georgie a list of healing habits to follow.

They were the same ones I used to help heal my body...

Healing habits to help awaken your body.

It is often the small things we consistently do that can have the greatest impact on our end results. Below is a practical set of healing habits I used to transform my daily patterns.

You can follow these healing habits for yourself or use them as the basis for creating your own. Remember to keep listening to your own body and do what works best for you.

1. Drink a big glass of lemon water upon arising.

2. Eat breakfast every day.

3. Eat real foods regularly throughout the day.

4. Eat high water content foods, especially leafy greens.

5. Increase protein in your diet (organic if possible).

6. Remove fake foods from your home and office.

7. Substitute fake foods with real foods.

8. Plan meals in advance for the week.

9. Schedule time for food shopping and preparation.

10. Season food with fresh herbs, lemon juice and sea salt.

11. Reduce artificial sweeteners and flavourings.

12. Reduce coffee or substitute it with a coffee-alternative.

13. Use high quality oils (organic if possible).

14. Do 5 minutes of gentle stretching before bed.

15. Take 3 deep breaths before eating.

Awakening your body.

Emotional eating is a way of silencing the messages that are coming from your body.

The key to transforming this dynamic is to identify what you are truly 'hungry' for.

The trouble for most women is that they were never taught how to listen or care for their bodies.

At the height of my emotional eating episodes, I felt totally disconnected from my body.

My mind ran the show.

I felt like I only existed from my shoulders upwards.

I was so focused upon my daily 'to-do' list'. I was convinced I didn't have time to listen to my body. Nor did I know how to, either.

My healing guide told me the antidote to silencing my body was listening to it instead.

"Are you saying I can actually ask my body for what it wants?"

"Yes of course" she said. *"You can communicate with your body any time you like!"*

Her words came as a complete surprise.

I lived in a culture that celebrated 'mind over matter'. It had never occurred to me that my body had its own intelligence.

I reflected back on all the times I had overridden my body. I had disregarded what it wanted or needed to feel healthy and happy.

I felt excited at the possibility of opening a dialogue with my body.

I couldn't wait to start experimenting...

Later that evening, I sat in my room to see if I could start communicating with my body.

I didn't know what to say.

So, I started with an apology.

Up until that point, it had only ever been a monologue, with my head shouting orders at my body.

In the beginning, our conversations were stunted.

I stayed committed to the process and focused on creating space for my body to express itself.

With time and practice my monologue began to transform into a dialogue between my head and my body.

As I befriended my body, it started to respond and express its' needs.

It shared with me that it was indeed hungry.

Not for the fake food that I thought it was craving.

Sometimes my body was dehydrated and it needed water.

Other times it felt starved of nutrients and it needed something nutritious to eat.

Or it was feeling sluggish and needed some gentle stretching and movement. Sometimes it was tired and in need of an early night.

When my life was too serious my body would tell me it needed more fun, relaxation and play.

When my body was feeling lonely, it would tell me it needed a hug. And reassurance that everything was going to be okay.

When you become aware of your emotional eating you can use it to understand what you are really hungry for.

Meeting up with Georgie a year later...

When I met up with Georgie a year later I couldn't believe the physical transformation that had taken place. She was brimming with energy.

"Wow! You look fabulous!" I said.

We hugged and I asked her how she had been.

"I am doing great" she replied. *"I have so much to tell you. Since I saw you last time, everything in my life has changed so much..."*

"After our session together, I started yoga. Practicing yoga helped me to become more aware of my body... It felt strange at first, but now, I love it!"

"That's super Georgie. What else have you been doing?"

"I started dialoguing with my body through my journal... I would take 15 minutes every morning to ask how it was feeling... And I actually listened for the answer... This helped me to rebuild my relationship with my body and make healthier choices."

"After slowly building my yoga practice, I focused upon breaking my addiction to sugar, especially chocolate..."

"That's wonderful!" I said. *"How did you do that?"*

"I substituted out all the bad things like processed foods, sugar and alcohol. I replaced them with good things. Like eating vegetables and leafy greens as well as drinking lots of water."

"I started doing it for a week as an experiment... The first few days were really difficult... I almost gave up... But I stuck with it... And I'm so glad that I did... By the seventh day I felt incredible... I started to wake up feeling energised and much more connected to my body too..."

"And Katrina, do you want to know an incredible thing?" she added.

"I've also met a lovely man. We've been dating for three months now... And I'm the healthiest and happiest I've felt in years!"

Your body knows the truth

"At times you have to leave the city of your comfort and go into the wilderness of your intuition. What you'll discover will be wonderful. What you'll discover is yourself."

~ Alan Alda

A number of years after I healed my emotional eating, I booked a one-way ticket to England. It included a month long stopover in Thailand.

When I was sick, tired and overweight the idea of being able to solo travel the world seemed impossible.

As the plane touched down on the tarmac, my heart was bursting with anticipation. My dream was becoming a reality.

Brimming with both nerves and excitement, I arrived in Bangkok with only my backpack.

I was staying right in the heart of Bangkok on Khao San Road. This central hub attracted travelers from all over the world.

The area was famous for its night markets and tantalising street food.

Sumptuous smells of fresh herbs and spices wafted along the ramshackle pavements.

Vendors would serve Thai delicacies straight from the flaming woks of their makeshift kitchens.

The flavor filled curries set fire to my taste buds. And the small parcels of sweet, sticky coconut rice soothed them.

After a week of sightseeing and eating my way through Bangkok, I was ready to move on to my next adventure.

I felt filled with possibility as I contemplated where to head next?

The hostel where I was staying was full of intrepid travellers. They were all trying to make the most of stretched pennies.

I wasn't sure of my next moves. So I thought the best thing to do would be to ask other people who knew Thailand better than I did.

I chatted to a lovely Danish couple who had travelled through Asia for three months.

They were on the tail end of their honeymoon and had spent most of their time in the North of Thailand.

When I shared with them I wasn't sure where to go next, they were emphatic I should head North to Chiang Mai. The newly-weds shared stories of a rich cultural landscape.

Stirred by their enthusiasm, I set off to a local café to research travel options online. I stumbled across some interesting looking yoga studios and Thai massage courses.

Once I had sketched a possible travel itinerary, I returned to my hostel.

At the reception area, I bumped into a bright and friendly girl from Australia. We were about the same age and discovered we had a shared passion for yoga and meditation.

I was inspired that she was a fellow solo traveller. She had spent six months traveling all over Thailand, Laos and Cambodia.

I asked her what she would do if she had 3 weeks left on her trip?

"If I was you, I would definitely head South."

She gushed about the turquoise waters and white sandy beaches. And also about drinking from green coconuts cut straight from the tree.

Our conversation dropped me into a dilemma...

Should I keep my sails set for the North as I had planned? Or should I change everything and let the winds take me South instead?

Knowing what to eat.

One of the biggest challenges on the healing journey is in knowing what to eat.

With so much contradictory information it can feel hard to make the right food choices. Everyone seems to have an opinion.

Some experts will advise you to eat plant-based vegetarian food. Others will insist on diets high in protein from meat, eggs and dairy. Some propose you should be eating all raw foods and others only cooked food.

Even scientific research studies often conflict with each other. It's a minefield for any woman who wants to feel happy and healthy.

When I was struggling with my health and weight challenges I was trying to eat what other people said I should eat.

The contradictory opinions of health experts left me in a state of confusion. Well-meaning friends and family only added to my frustration. I didn't know who to follow or trust.

I shared my predicament with my healing guide.

"Katrina, the thing most diet books don't tell you is that your body is the ultimate authority" she said. *"It is the thing you should be paying attention to above all else."*

"Are you saying my body knows more than all the experts out there?" I asked.

"Yes that's right. Have you ever seen an animal consult a diet book?" she chuckled. *"Of course not, they instinctively know what to eat".*

"Katrina, you are the one living inside your body. You must learn to listen and attune to its unique rhythm and needs. Most women have been taught to distrust their natural instincts... And this is why they struggle... It was never meant to be this way..."

Her words reverberated through me. It was a powerful revelation...

Choosing the right fuel for your body.

"How do I know what food to eat?" I asked my healing guide.

"Katrina the best way to know what to eat is by paying attention to your body's unique feedback."

"It's important to be aware your body has its own language. It is always speaking to you... The trouble is you haven't been listening."

"When you nourish your body with proper nutrition, it will bless you with energy, health and well being. When you deprive your body it will respond with cravings, lethargy and illness."

"I have never thought of it that way before." I replied. *"I guess my body is telling me I haven't been treating it so well..."*

"Katrina, that's a powerful thing to realise" she said.

"You can build upon this awareness by noticing how your body feels before, during and after eating. Look for feelings of heaviness, bloating, indigestion, reflux, constipation and weight gain."

"Oh, I experience all those things," I replied.

"Well this is a sign you are eating food your body is struggling to process."

"Wow, that's so interesting..." I said.

"Katrina, common foods that cause discomfort and inflammation are gluten, dairy, sugar, caffeine and alcohol..." she said.

"Once you identify trouble foods, you can substitute them with foods that are easier to digest."

"Easing the strain on your digestive track will support your body to process the foods you eat."

"This will help to cleanse and strengthen your digestive system. It will also help you to rebuild your immune system."

Listening to the intuitive guidance of my body.

I returned back to Bangkok from the North of Thailand.

My body had given me the intuitive guidance to visit Chiang Mai so I decided to stick to my original plan.

The whole trip had been a big step outside of my comfort zone.

I enrolled in the Thai massage course and discovered new ways of connecting with and moving my body. I made friends from around the world and hired a motorbike for the first time. I also swam in a pristine pool of spring water underneath a waterfall. It was magical.

I crossed the border into Laos and visited its lively capital Vientiane. I loved all the French-colonial architecture, Buddhist temples and Euro-Asian inspired cuisine.

On the day I was due to depart for England, my body gave me an unusual message... *"Delay your flight and head South."*

It seemed like an insane idea. My mind immediately disregarded it.

As I ate a fresh tropical fruit salad for breakfast, my body wouldn't let up. It insisted it wasn't ready to head to London yet. Instead it yearned to spend a few weeks relaxing in a hammock on a beach in the South of Thailand.

I called the airline to see if could postpone my flight. I anticipated it would be either too late or too expensive.

To my surprise, the customer support person informed me I could make one flight change *"free of charge"*.

I couldn't believe my luck. I hung up the phone and clapped my hands in delight. It dawned on me I didn't have to choose between the North or South of Thailand, as I had thought.

By having the courage to listen to the wisdom of my body, I was able to give myself the precious gift of visiting both...

Chapter summary.

Overriding your body comes from being unaware of its true needs.

Fake energy can come from coffee, sugar, soda, fake food, alcohol and even certain drugs.

Real energy comes from drinking clean water and eating real foods.

It also comes from gently moving your body, spending time in nature and having good sleep patterns.

Awakening your body begins the moment you start paying attention to its unique needs.

You can start by asking your body whether it enjoys the foods you are eating?

Begin to notice how you feel after you eat certain foods.

Are you savouring and enjoying the taste of your food?

What happens when you combine different foods? Do you experience any discomfort, bloating or pain?

You can dialogue with your body by keeping a journal. Regularly check in with it and keep asking what it needs to be healthy and happy.

The idea is not to become perfect but to make progress every day.

Remember that your body knows the truth. Real healing happens when you honour its innate wisdom.

When you show deep care for your body it will reward you with feelings of vibrant health and wellness.

It will also reveal how miraculous it is.

Chapter Eight – Connect With Your Emotions

"Notice what happens when you doubt, suppress, or act contrary to your feelings. You will observe decreased energy, powerless or helpless feelings, and physical or emotional pain. Now notice what happens when you follow your intuitive feelings. Usually the result is increased energy and power and a sense of natural flow. When you're at one with yourself, the world feels peaceful, exciting, and magical."

~ Shakti Gawain

Notice emotional pain

"For me, singing sad songs often has a way of healing a situation. It gets the hurt out in the open into the light, out of the darkness."

~ Reba McEntire

I was 12 years old when I started gymnastics.

I was in my first year of secondary school and beginning a new chapter in my life.

I had spent my primary years attending a small school in a rural farming community. There was one head principal, two teachers and 25 wide-eyed country kids.

My high school had closer to 500 students. With no elder siblings to guide me, I had to navigate this vast new realm on my own.

I still remember the first day I caught the school bus. I sat alone feeling scared and unsure of myself in the presence of older children.

Our school uniform was unflattering. It consisted of a thick woollen tartan kilt, plain white shirt and a pea green V-neck jumper.

Wearing it made me feel embarrassed and uncomfortable. It also made me feel self-conscious about my body and appearance for the first time.

My new school offered an after-school curriculum of activities.

I signed up for a gymnastics class having no idea what to expect. Much to my surprise, I found I enjoyed it. It was fun and I soon began to develop physical strength, confidence and new friendships.

One day our coach announced a special gymnastics event was going to be held in our town. She informed us we would each need to undergo an audition before the final teams were selected.

I had no idea what an audition was but it sounded exciting...

The announcement created a sense of anticipation in our gym class.

The girls pursued their routines with a new vigour. Their enthusiasm stirred something within me and I vowed to rise to the occasion.

The week after the auditions our coach announced she had selected the final teams. Rather than read the names out loud, she pinned them to the noticeboard by the change rooms.

We didn't need any further encouragement. Our troupe of giddy giggling girls rushed over to read the list.

I scanned through the names but I couldn't see mine anywhere.

I read through the 'A' team... the 'B' team... the 'C' team...

Something was wrong. I re-read the list, only this time more carefully.

I saw the names of friends from gym class. But I didn't see mine.

Then one girl shrieked, *"Katrina, you're in the D-Team!"*

All the other girls cackled hysterically.

I read on in disbelief until I finally saw my name.

She was right. I had been placed in the 'D' team.

But not only that, I had been nominated as the Captain.

I had officially been selected as 'the best of the worst'.

It was devastating.

My cheeks flushed with the hue of humiliation.

I felt like a crystal bowl knocked onto a concrete floor. My self-confidence shattered into a million pieces.

My eyes welled with tears and I scurried away to the change rooms...

Physical wounds versus emotional wounds.

Growing up can be difficult.

As we develop we all undergo a series of tests, trials and tribulations.

These can often result in physical and emotional wounds that create pain in our lives.

Physical wounds can be protected with plasters, bandages and casts whilst the body heals.

Our cuts, scrapes and bruises are readily detectable to the naked eye, making them relatively easy to tend to.

Emotional wounds are more obscure. They exist in the subtle realm of our inner world, making them harder to identify and care for.

Emotional wounds can result from painful experiences that induce uncomfortable feelings. Such as fear, anxiety, guilt, shame, embarrassment, rejection, sadness, loneliness, despair and grief.

Early life experiences can imprint upon a child. It can leave them feeling unworthy, undeserving and unlovable as adults.

Most children don't have the maturity or tools to tend to their emotional wounds. As a result they rarely heal fully.

Life events push, prod and poke these emotional wounds amplifying the hurt.

These wounds create the need for relief through coping strategies like emotional eating. It can also create the unconscious desire for protection through weight gain.

Layer by layer our 'emotional scar tissue' builds upon itself.

Eventually the emotional pain becomes too much to endure.

This is the signal that the healing journey is ready to begin.

My first summer holiday job.

"Katrina, can you come in tomorrow at 4pm for a staff training?"

"Yes." I replied.

"Great, we'll see you then…" said my new manager.

I was 15 years old and I had just landed myself a holiday job. It was in a busy bakery in a popular tourist town in New Zealand.

Over the summer months this resort town would swell to the brim with holidaymakers.

There were ten teenage girls starting work that day. We all assembled in the customer service area of the bakery.

The manager announced the first thing she needed to do was to assign us work uniforms.

She then escorted us into a storeroom and closed the door behind us.

The room was hot, stuffy and smelt like fermented sour dough.

A solitary bulb swung from the ceiling dimly lighting the space.

Industrial storage shelves with cage like metal framing covered the walls.

Each shelf was packed full of the bits of the baking business. There were boxes of tea, coffee, serviettes, packaging, labels and signage all jammed in.

With measuring tape in hand, my manager asked us to form an orderly line. I did what I was told and filed in towards the end.

I took a closer look at the girls standing around me and couldn't help but compare myself to them.

They all seemed taller than me. Much skinnier and prettier too…

One by one the girls were measured. They were then handed a crisp white uniform, folded maroon apron and a pleated bakers hat.

Perspiration seeped from my forehead as I waited my turn.

Perhaps there was still time for me to sneak away?

"Katrina, can you please step forward?" my manager said.

All eyes in the room locked down on me.

I felt all sweaty and exposed.

I sucked in my tummy and stumbled forward.

My manager asked me to extend my hands out to the side. She then used her tape to measure me around the bust, waist, hips and arms.

She wrote down my measurements in her notepad. She then began rummaging inside a black plastic box that contained the uniforms.

Looking perplexed, she asked if she could measure me again?

Bust... waist... hips... arms...

There was more ruffling. She then announced,

"Katrina, we don't appear to have any uniforms in your size."

I was mortified.

Indifferent to my escalating embarrassment, she added,

"Don't worry dear... I'll order a larger sized uniform in especially for you... It should arrive early next week..."

I could hear the other girls snorting behind me. And it hurt.

In that moment I wished I could shrink into a tiny fleck of dust and disappear from sight...

Understanding emotional pain.

Women book *Breakthrough Healing Sessions* with me when they are in emotional pain.

Many of my clients say they feel stuck, blocked or restricted in some area of their life.

They know life could be so much more fun and enjoyable. Yet they feel burdened by something that is preventing them from moving forward.

Many find themselves turning to a coping strategy like emotional eating to get by. And I can understand why. I longed for a sweeter existence that only seemed attainable through food.

As a healer, I have found that the roots of emotional pain are nearly always seeded in childhood.

During a session a client will often trace back to an emotional wound from their formative years.

A child's sense of emotional wellbeing is strongly influenced by their early experiences.

Through punishment and reward a child learns which emotions are safe to express. They then adopt strategies to win attention, acceptance and affection.

As open and empathic beings they absorb the emotional energy from their surroundings.

These early childhood experiences mold a child's sense of self and worldview. They can also establish patterns of behaviour that can last well into adulthood.

Taking time to explore these early childhood dynamics can help build greater self-awareness.

It can also provide insight into the kinds of emotions that trigger emotional eating.

Emotional pain gets stored within the physical body.

As adults, we call in people and life experiences to remind us of what remains unhealed within us. If we allow ourselves to see beyond the surface level drama, we can identify our next level of healing.

One thing I discovered was that my unresolved emotional pain didn't go away on its own. Regardless of how much I wished it would.

Emotional pain gets stored in our physical bodies. It remains here until we are better able to process and release it.

Even though emotional pain gets stored in the body, it doesn't have to remain there. You can use healing tools to help move this old emotional residue out of your body.

Just as your wardrobe needs regular clearing and updating, so too does your emotional world.

You can expand your emotional bandwidth beyond the pain and hurt you have suffered. It begins with a willingness to align your emotional programs with who you are and what you value today.

You can start releasing old emotional energy by experimenting with different healing tools. Try massage, yoga, essential oils, flower remedies and emotional freedom technique (EFT).

Seek out therapists, teachers and healing guides that you feel safe with and can trust. Ask your intuition to guide you in the right direction.

When you do your inner healing work, you remove the charge of your old emotions.

As you release and heal them, you will find they no longer hold any power over you. You will also notice your desire for emotional eating will dissolve.

I have seen the most stunning transformations in my *Breakthrough Healing Sessions.* When clients release old memories from their bodies they say they feel lighter and more at peace.

Exercise: What emotions trigger your emotional eating?

Use the following checklist to build your awareness of the kinds of emotions that trigger your emotional eating...

Tick the feelings that feel true for you...

I emotionally eat when I feel...	Yes / No	I emotionally eat when I feel...	Yes / No
Afraid		Powerless	
Angry		Rejected	
Ashamed		Resistant	
Awkward		Sad	
Bitter		Spiteful	
Bored		Stressed	
Depressed		Stuck	
Distracted		Tired	
Embarrassed		Trapped	
Exhausted		Unappreciated	
Frustrated		Undeserving	
Happy		Unimportant	
Hurt		Unsafe	
Jealous		Upset	
Judged		Unworthy	

Release stuck emotions

"Negative emotions like loneliness, envy, and guilt have an important role to play in a happy life; they're big, flashing signs that something needs to change..."

~ Gretchen Rubin

As Helen lay down on my healing table she began sobbing.

I began our *Breakthrough Healing Session* by reassuring her that she was in the right place. And that everything was going to be okay.

Helen was a teacher struggling with emotional eating. She had been suppressing her emotions with food and was ready for a shift.

As she lay on the table I invited her to close her eyes.

I guided her to breathe into her heart and allow her body to soften and relax.

I then proceeded to do some gentle healing work until she was calm and able to speak comfortably...

"Katrina, I don't know if I should have come to see you today... I feel so uncomfortable... Just awful and bloated... I've been eating chocolate to make myself feel better. And then I feel so angry with myself afterwards. I don't know what to do anymore... I feel totally stuck..."

Helen covered her face with her hands.

"It seems like nothing in my life is ever going to change... Or if it does, it's only going to get worse..."

I invited Helen to take another deep breath and notice the support of the table underneath her...

I assured her the more she was able to trust and let go of the past, the deeper the healing process would be...

"Helen, where does this feeling live inside your body?" I asked.

"This feeling is everywhere... It starts out as a heaviness inside my chest and then it seeps into the rest of my body..."

"Does this feeling have a colour or texture?" I asked.

"Yes it's dark... And it feels all gluggy... And, it's covering over everything inside me... It feels like a thick, sticky mud..." she said.

"And if this thick, sticky mud had an emotion, what would it be?"

"Katrina, I feel like it is all my fears and doubts. I feel so uncertain and unclear about what I'm doing with my life at the moment."

"And how does this uncertainty affect you?" I enquired.

"Pretty much everywhere" she replied. *"I feel afraid in so many areas of my life... Especially at work... But, also at home... It feels like all my hopes and dreams are buried deep inside of me. And I am scared that they will never see the light of day..."*

"Helen you are doing great..." I said.

"Katrina, I constantly feel as if time is passing me by. I worry that I'm leaving it too late... What if something happens to me? What if I get sick? Or my husband does? What if I never get to travel? Or have time to do the things I've always dreamed of doing?"

"All this worry leaves me feeling scared and anxious... I then turn to food to take these dreadful feelings away..."

"And if you could give this feeling a rating, where 'one' is nothing and 'ten' is very intense, what would it be?" I asked.

"It's off the scales ... I'd call it an eleven or twelve."

We had our starting point.

Now it was time to see if Helen's stuck emotions were ready to release from her body…

Stuck emotions versus flowing emotions.

In my *Breakthrough Healing Sessions*, I help women to transform stuck emotional patterns.

Your emotions are a powerful energy source and are designed to move freely. You can think of the word 'e-motion' translating to 'energy in motion'. However like a river it is possible for this natural flow to become blocked, impeded or stuck.

Stuck emotions can manifest as fear, frustration, anger, disappointment, bitterness and depression. These emotions can become trapped inside the body and can drain your life force energy.

Stuck emotions emerge out of our unaddressed emotional pain. They can also come from rigid beliefs about how 'life is' or 'should be'.

As children we learn that certain emotions are bad, negative or shameful. This often sets up a desire to shun, suppress or disown these feelings rather than express them.

Stuck emotions can make you feel frustrated, overwhelmed and unable to make changes. They can also trigger emotional eating.

All stuck emotions are waiting to be transformed into flowing emotions.

Flowing emotions are your natural state of being. They manifest as growth, happiness, luck, opportunity, synchronicity, abundance, blessings and good fortune.

When you allow yourself to feel and express your emotions, you can release them from your body.

Allowing your feelings to move in a flowing way, cultivates emotional wellbeing. This can help balance your life without a coping strategy like emotional eating.

Through this sacred enquiry you can cultivate a deeper connection with yourself. It will also open the door to helping you experience more health, happiness and joy in your life.

Transforming stuck emotions into flowing emotions.

When I work with clients, I like to invite them to notice whether their emotions feel stuck or flowing.

Unconscious patterns are often inaccessible to the rational part of the brain. This can make them tricky to recognise and deal with.

This is why women can find themselves eating foods they know are not good for them. It also explains why the dieting model fails in practice for most women.

Our unconscious mind works in a different way to our logical mind.

Like our dream world, it reveals itself in colours, pictures, patterns, shapes, shades, sounds, smells, symbols and textures.

In my sessions, I help my clients gain a glimpse of how their unconscious mind processes the world.

I do this by inviting them to notice how their emotions feel within their bodies. Most clients share vivid descriptions of the imagery they see.

Through my healing work I have discovered that these inner configurations are malleable.

Once a client can describe how their stuck emotions feel, we begin the process of moving the energy. I assist in this process by using gentle healing tools. Such as tapping, energy work, guided meditation, breathing techniques and healing affirmations.

As the energy moves, so too do my clients internal representations.

The stuck energy morphs into new images and patterns. The associated feelings also transform becoming much lighter, expansive and flowing.

Releasing stuck emotions can help you to break old patterns. And as a result give you the ability to make new empowering choices.

It will also help you to *Heal Emotional Eating For Good.*

Moving stuck energy.

I started gently tapping on different energetic points on Helen's body, to see if her stuck energy was ready to move.

As I was tapping, I asked Helen *"If you could speak to your doubts what would you say to them?"*

"Let go of me!" she replied. *"I'm sick and tired of you holding me back..."*

"Okay, that's a great starting point" I said. *"But what if your doubts were just trying to get your attention? What happens when you turn around and face them instead?"*

Helen fell silent...

"Katrina, it never occurred to me I could face my doubts before. It always seemed so much easier to try and run away from them..."

"And what do you notice now that you are facing them?" I asked.

"Well they are not as scary as I thought... They appear all soft and fluffy... Like stuffed toys... It seems a bit ridiculous to be running from them."

"Yes" I replied. *"Often our doubts are just smaller parts of us crying out for love and understanding..."*

We carried on with our tapping and energetic release work...

Towards the end of our *Breakthrough Healing Session* I asked Helen to close her eyes and check in with her body.

"Katrina, it's amazing. All the thick, sticky mud has completely disappeared. It isn't there anymore. And I feel so much lighter too."

Helen was radiating an inner strength, joy and peacefulness.

She left the healing session beaming like a warm summer day...

Exercise: Releasing your stuck emotions.

Stuck emotions live inside your body just waiting to be recognised and released.

A powerful way to release them is through 'tapping'.

This involves gently tapping on different meridian points to move the energy. It's one of the healing tools I use in my *Breakthrough Healing Sessions.*

The main tapping points are…

(i) top of the head

(ii) along the eyebrow

(iii) on the checkbone

(iv) under the nose

(v) on the chin

(vi) across the collar bone

(vii) rib cage on the side of the body

(viii) side of the hand

Preparation for the tapping session:

Drink a glass of water before and after the session.

Create a sacred space where you know you won't be disturbed. Set aside at least 20 minutes. Keep a pen and paper handy so you can write down any insights you receive.

Take some deep breaths with slow inhalations and long exhalations.

Close your eyes if you wish and set a healing intention.

Instructions:

1. Bring awareness to your body.

2. Focus on emotional eating or a specific food you crave.

3. Scan your body and notice:

(a) Where is the feeling located in your body?

(b) Does the feeling have a colour?

(c) Does the feeling have a shape?

(d) Does the feeling have a texture?

(e) What size is the feeling?

(f) How intense is the feeling? Give it a rating from 1-10.

4. Start tapping on different meridian points of your body.

Repeat short phrases such as 'this feeling', 'my cravings' and 'my emotional eating' and notice what comes up for you.

5. Let yourself feel your feelings. Old emotional energy can release through crying, yawning and even laughter.

6. Keep tapping on the meridian points until the intensity reduces and the feeling subsides.

7. As the feeling releases, move, stretch and shake your body.

8. Journal any guidance you receive.

9. If you feel tired after tapping give yourself permission to rest.

Embrace self-expression

"The thing that is really hard, and really amazing, is giving up on being perfect and beginning the work of becoming yourself."

~ Anna Quindlen

Alice was attending one of my *Yoga and Healing Retreats*.

She booked a *Breakthrough Healing Session* with me to work on her emotional eating.

When she arrived in my healing room, I asked if she would like to share a little more with me...

"Katrina, my emotional eating is ruining my life..." she said.

"I've been too ashamed to speak about this to anyone... I'm at my wits end and really don't know what else I can do... I hope you don't mind me sharing this with you... I thought you might understand what I am going through..."

"The thing is I can't stop my cravings, or my obsessive compulsive thoughts about food. The more I try to control my eating, the more it controls me..."

"I'm worried I might be addicted to potato crisps. I can't stop thinking about them. Each time I open a new packet, I promise myself I will only eat a handful..."

"But, as soon as the dry salty flavor of that first chip dissolves in my mouth... Something comes over me. I become a different person... and I just can't stop myself..."

"Before I know it, I've devoured the whole pack..."

"Can you recommend a diet that will help me?"

"Alice, before we dive into possible solutions, can you tell me what else is happening in your life?"

"Well Katrina, I have so much to be grateful for..."

"I'm happily single which gives me a lot of freedom over my spare time... I live in a nice flat... And I have lovely connections with my friends and family as well..."

"That's really great Alice..." I said. *"Now is there anything in your life that isn't going quite as well as you would like?"*

"Mmm... I guess that would be my job..." she said.

Alice shared that she worked at an advertising agency.

"Katrina, I felt so blessed when I started my job... The whole thing seemed to fall into my lap..."

"Everything was so new and exciting... The travel, the people and all the amazing parties... All my friends told me how lucky I was..."

"But, lately I find myself dreading going into work..."

"I'm normally a really positive person but the daily grind is starting to get me down. Especially the long hours, the boring meetings and office politics..."

"Is there something else you would like to be doing instead?" I asked.

"Oh, I don't know, Katrina... Really, I don't..." she sighed.

"Okay, Alice... What if I was to say you had full permission to do whatever you wanted. Is there something you would love to do?"

"Anything? Absolutely anything at all?"

"Yes, anything you like..." I replied.

"Hmmm... Well... I would love to be able to sing all day long..."

"Super" I said. *"Have you ever considered doing that?"*

"Doing what?" she asked.

"Sing all day long..." I said.

"Sing all day long? You mean me... Sing all day long? Like... for a living...?"

"Yes" I replied. *"Lots of people do."*

"Katrina, there's no way that I could do that... I mean that would be ridiculous... What would I do for money? How would I pay my rent? And, what about my bills?"

"Why would you even suggest that?" she asked.

"Well Alice, as soon as you spoke about singing all day long I felt a surge of life force energy pulse through your body. It was palpable."

"Really? You felt that?"

"Yes," I said.

"Katrina, I would love for my whole life to be based around singing... but my mind tells me I should be sensible..."

"I go round and round in circles hoping my life could be different. But then convincing myself that it is going to stay like this forever."

"And then this dark and helpless feeling descends over me. And that is when I reach for food to take that awful feeling away..."

We had arrived at a truth point.

I invited Alice to take a nice long deep breath into her heart.

I sensed that an old emotional program was ready to release.

And a new possibility was ready to be born...

Emotional suppression versus emotional expression.

Many clients ask me how they can manage their emotions more effectively in their lives.

Rather than try to manage their emotions, what I encourage them to do is express them instead.

What I have discovered is emotional energy can either move 'destructively' or 'creatively'.

Trying to manage how you feel can often trigger destructive emotional eating tendencies.

This can also happen to women who try to control their cravings through dieting.

Women who diet without addressing the root cause usually end up sabotaging their best efforts.

The alternative is to learn how to express your emotional energy in a creative way instead.

Learning how to express my emotional energy in a creative way had a transformative affect on my life.

You can try this out for yourself by experimenting with different creative practices. Take time to identify and explore ones that feel fun and joyful for you.

Experiment with dancing, singing, sculpting, painting, drawing, writing, decorating, designing, sewing, gardening or travelling.

The key to healing is to channel your vital life force energy away from your addictions. And towards the realisation of your dreams.

After our *Breakthrough Healing Session* Alice allowed singing to play a larger role in her life.

By listening to her heart she transformed her emotional eating. She now shares her passion for singing with others…

Chapter summary.

On your healing journey, you have the opportunity to release emotional programs you have outgrown.

Your emotions are a powerful force waiting to be directed towards your dreams.

You don't have to live your life being constrained or limited by your stuck emotions any longer.

It begins by tending to the emotional wounds you have endured along the way.

Emotional energy always wants to move. And it will move either in a creative or destructive direction.

As you connect with your emotions, you can heal your old wounds and release any stuck emotional programs.

Pay attention to your pain and let it catalyse you into the woman you are truly capable of becoming.

When emotions are suppressed, energy becomes stuck. This can create drama, difficulty and despair.

There is a creative power sitting dormant within you. You can choose to activate this potent force whenever you feel ready.

Give yourself permission to make new choices in your life. When you choose to express your emotions in healthy ways you can start to create the life of your dreams.

This will allow you to live a creatively self-expressed and inspired life.

One filled with adventure, health, happiness, fun, laughter and play.

Chapter Nine – Change Your Stories

"It's like everyone tells a story about themselves inside their own head. Always. All the time. That story makes you what you are. We build ourselves out of that story."

~ Patrick Rothfuss

Become aware of your stories

"The greatest weapon against stress is our ability to choose one thought over another."

~ William James

As I read the newspaper advertisement, I felt my body tremble with an unusual kind of trepidation.

There written in black and white print was an invitation to join an 8-day adventure camp in the New Zealand wilderness.

I was 28 years old and at a key transition point in my life. I had some important decisions to make and was in need of a little inspiration.

Perhaps some time in nature would help bring clarity?

I wasn't convinced but was curious to find out more.

I read through the website and familiarised myself with the ethos of the camp and its course leaders. I also skimmed through the glowing array of testimonials from past participants...

And it all sounded great. Really it did.

My main concern was around the physical activities. I was hardly the 'outdoors type' and was worried the experience might be too demanding for me.

Would I be able to keep up? What if I wanted to opt out of one or more of the activities? Would they publicly mock or ridicule me?

Or call me a wimp?

After considerable deliberation, I came to the conclusion the camp wasn't for me.

I felt pleased with my decision and did my best to forget all about it...

Over the next few days, the spirit of the camp kept sending little signs to let me know it wasn't ready to give up on me.

Like a catchy pop song, it kept sneaking back into my mind when I least expected it.

One night I even dreamt I was fireside, toasting marshmallows under a clear moonlit sky.

I returned back to the website to make sure there wasn't something I had missed.

To my surprise I discovered the camp offered part scholarships. This was to assist young people who didn't have the means to pay full price.

My eyebrows pricked up. Maybe I could do this?

I applied on a whim, fully expecting to be rejected. I figured it would be the easiest way to bring the matter to an end.

A couple of weeks later, I received a letter awarding me a bursary.

I was stunned. Perhaps it was destined to be?

The first day of camp arrived all too soon.

There were 12 participants in all. We were an oddly assembled troupe of different ages, interests and backgrounds. The one thing we shared was an uncertainty about what the camp would bring.

Each day we were given a range of different activities to take part in. They included orienteering, rock climbing, canoeing and sailing.

Each activity was designed to push us beyond our comfort zones.

We also learnt valuable life skills like teamwork, leadership, vision, communication and persistence.

I was stretching every cell within my body and I was achieving things I never thought possible...

On day five, my newfound zeal was dealt a sobering blow…

I was one of the last to return to camp after an early morning hike. I had scraped my knee and blood blisters had appeared on the soles of my feet. I felt defeated and was on the brink of quitting.

Back at base camp there was no time for my whining and whimpering.

Our team leader called us all together. He then barked that we had 30 minutes to prepare for our ultimate challenge… *'Solo'*.

Solo was a two-night wilderness mission we had to complete alone.

I gasped with fright.

Our leader was strong and sinewy like a mountain goat. I looked at him with utter disbelief. A voice inside my head squawked…

"Live alone in the wild? Surely he must be joking? I can't be expected to do this? I'm a young woman, not a hardened survivalist…"

He informed us we would each be given a piece of rope and a black plastic tarp to construct a basic shelter.

Before I could muster my protest speech, I was handed a canteen of drinking water and a brown paper ration bag.

The bag contained three carrots, two apples and an oatmeal cookie. It seemed barely enough to feed a small rabbit let alone sustain my life.

I swallowed hard as I imagined living out my own apocalypse.

Our camp leader explained that *Solo* would challenge us all in our own unique ways. He told us to journal our thoughts and feelings, as it would give us valuable insights about our lives.

As a parting gift, he asked us to contemplate the following question…

"What would you do with your life if you weren't so afraid?"

I silently whispered to myself, *"Refuse to sleep alone in the wild!"*

Becoming aware of your stories.

To *Heal Emotional Eating For Good* it is important to become aware of the stories you tell yourself.

In particular, the painful stories you regularly repeat and accept as truth.

Our stories are the internal narratives we construct to make sense of our lives. They incorporate our beliefs and affect our perceptions. These stories filter the way we view the world.

The old and outdated stories we tell ourselves can inhibit us from living the life we are capable of.

Humans are imaginative and have the ability to create stories about all sorts of things. We weave stories about life events, other people and ourselves to create a sense of meaning.

We use stories to explain our relationship to food, friends, family, love, money, exercise, health, as well as our bodies.

Our stories affect our future possibilities by influencing what we allow ourselves to do.

The foundations of our stories are laid in childhood. They are influenced from the narratives we hear from the outside world. They are also affected by our own unique life experiences.

We progressively build upon our stories into adulthood as we solidify the way that we see the world.

Once we have constructed our stories, we gather evidence to support them. We surround ourselves with people who validate our stories. And we also tend to dismiss anything that may disprove them.

Our stories become more hypnotic each time we tell them. They can become so 'spellbinding' that we rarely stop to question them.

Through dramatisation and selective revision our stories can often bear little resemblance to reality.

Becoming aware of my stories.

Many of the stories I would tell myself I had authored as a child. As I grew older, it didn't occur to me I could revise and update them.

These stories would often create stressful feelings that would influence my food choices. When the feelings were intense enough they would also trigger my emotional eating patterns.

What made it challenging was the fact I didn't even know I was telling myself stories.

I had always assumed the things I would repeatedly tell myself were indicative of 'how life was'. I was convinced of the validity of my stories and believed them without question.

I gathered all sorts of 'evidence' to prove their legitimacy. Regardless of the angst this would cause me. Believing my painful stories would leave me reaching for 'fake food' to feel better.

Once I had chosen to heal, I started to become aware of the different kinds of stories I would tell myself.

Although things were pretty foggy at first, a new sense of clarity began to emerge.

I could see that much of the pain in my life was created by the stories I was telling myself and not from pain itself.

I found I not only had the power to observe my stories but also question them as well.

I began to identify the thoughts that would invoke my resistance and self-sabotage patterns.

All I had to do was pay attention to my stories and notice the emotions they would create.

This awareness was liberating and gave me the courage to step forward on my healing journey.

Stories I used to tell myself.

Below is a selection of stories I would tell myself that would trigger my emotional eating. Can you relate to any of them?

"My life is so hard..."

"Nobody listens to me..."

"I don't fit in..."

"It's not fair..."

"I'm not good enough..."

"I shouldn't have eaten that..."

"Food is my worst enemy..."

"I'm different to other people..."

"My body is always letting me down..."

"I don't know what to do..."

"I never get to have any fun..."

"My life is such a struggle..."

"I've tried everything..."

"I'll never lose weight..."

"People are always taking advantage of me..."

"I never want to feel hurt again..."

"I never get to do what I want..."

"My life is never going to change..."

Journaling is a powerful healing tool.

One of the healing tools I use to become aware of my stories is the practice of journaling.

Journaling can help you to generate new insights in all areas of your life. Including your emotional eating patterns.

I discovered the power of journaling when I started my healing journey.

My healing guide recommended I create a food journal to build awareness of my eating habits.

This inspired me to create a personal *Healing Journal.* This was so I could write down all the foods I was eating.

I later expanded my journal to include writing about my thoughts and feelings. I would do this for 10-15 minutes each day.

Even though my early journaling attempts were pretty basic, I still found the process useful.

It gave me the chance to become more real and honest with myself. It provided me with a sacred space to connect with the feelings that I was too afraid to share with anyone else.

Expressing my inner rumblings helped me to witness the stories I had been telling myself.

It also helped me to see the connection between my thoughts, feelings and food cravings.

The process of journaling is so illuminating that I still use it to this day.

Journaling is a great healing tool to try out as you progress along your journey. It's particularly useful when you are at the edge of your comfort zone and ready for a breakthrough.

It will provide you with the insight to move beyond the stories that drive your emotional eating.

Exercise: Developing your journaling practice.

You can build awareness of your stories by developing your own journaling practice.

Begin by writing down your thoughts and feelings on blank paper for 10 minutes a day.

Journaling will help you identify the inner dialogue triggering your emotional eating.

This can include the stories that you tell yourself. As well as the people, places and situations in your life that cause you unnecessary stress.

It will allow you to become more aware of your stories and how they affect your eating habits and food choices.

As you journal, there is no need to censor what you write. Nor concern yourself with grammar, punctuation or spelling.

Simply put your pen to paper and give yourself permission to write from your heart.

The great thing with this healing tool is that you can journal anytime in the day that suits you. I find mornings work best for me.

Instructions:

Choose somewhere comfortable to journal. Make sure it is a place where you will be free from potential distractions or interruptions.

Take 10 minutes to write about your life and how you are feeling. This can include any stress or pain you are experiencing as well as your food choices.

Aim to write about 2-3 pages using blank paper.

Repeat this journaling practice daily for the next 21 days and be open and curious to what you discover.

Transform your disempowering stories

"Healing may not be so much about getting better, as about letting go of everything that isn't you - all of the expectations, all of the beliefs - and becoming who you are."

~ Rachel Naomi Remen

Stephanie booked a *Breakthrough Healing Session* while on a *Yoga and Healing Retreat* with me.

She was a bubbly, sensitive and caring woman who worked for a charity.

She had been struggling with emotional eating for a number of years.

Stephanie confided she had been nervous about coming to see me.

She had never had a healing session before and was worried about what it might bring up for her.

"There is absolutely nothing to be afraid of..." I said.

"You are in a safe space and we will only work with the thoughts and feelings that are ready to release naturally..."

"Katrina, I have to admit it feels so strange for me to be reaching out for help. I've always been the kind of person other people turn to. So this is a new experience for me..."

"The truth is, I've never felt comfortable revealing my emotions to others. It's like I keep my real feelings hidden inside of me."

Stephanie straightened as she wished away her tears.

"Ohh Katrina, I won't allow myself to cry... Not even now".

"Stephanie all of our emotions want to move freely. Particularly the ones we've been trying to suppress for so long..."

"Can I ask how you deal with difficult and uncomfortable feelings?"

"Katrina, I use food to make myself feel better. And alcohol too... And sometimes it works... But then it doesn't... And lately it hardly seems to be working at all... It all feels so loathsome... It's like being sucked down into a spiraling whirlpool I can't pull myself out of..."

"And where does this feeling live inside your body?" I asked.

"My throat... It's all trapped in my throat..." she said. *"It feels red. Inflamed. It's like it's all raw, tight and constricted."*

"You are doing great Stephanie. Now if there was an emotion attached to your throat what would it be?"

"Katrina I'd have to say anger. The feeling is anger..."

"Does this surprise you?" I asked.

"Yes it does. I've never seen myself as an angry type of person."

"And how does it feel to be holding this anger in your throat?"

"It's awful..." she said. *"It feels like I've been holding on to the words I've been too afraid to speak my entire life... And it's become so painful... I've been using food to try and push down these feelings..."*

"And Stephanie, how is this affecting you?"

"Katrina, it's depressing... And dark... It feels like I'm under this constant pressure to hold everything together... Whatever happens and whatever the costs... I have to be strong and never show my emotions publicly... Or any kind of vulnerability... Or weakness... Even when I'm hurting inside."

"And it's dead lonely... I don't feel as if I have anyone in my life I can turn to. No one seems to understand me. Not even my family or closest friends..."

Empowering stories versus disempowering stories.

I like to share with my clients that our stories can be either 'empowering' or 'disempowering'.

Empowering stories inspire our greatness. They can create a sense of fun, adventure, clarity and a desire to move forward.

They are narrated with the voice of encouragement, kindness, compassion, curiosity and possibility.

Empowering stories give you the courage to step beyond your perceived limitations. They provide the strength necessary to overcome any obstacle you may encounter.

These stories are aligned with our true nature. They propel us forward in the direction of our dreams and highest aspirations.

Empowering stories attract opportunities, synchronicity, joy, flow and feelings of abundance. They will also give you the inner conviction necessary to *Heal Emotional Eating For Good.*

Disempowering stories keep us stuck in the past. Living within the confines of our comfort zones. They hold us back from confronting our fears and inhibitions.

They are narrated with the voice of fear, frustration, criticism, uncertainty and limitation.

Disempowering stories can leave you feeling powerless to make positive change.

These stories can create self-sabotage patterns. And keep you stuck living from your smaller self.

We tell ourselves disempowering stories to reduce the risk of looking foolish, getting hurt or being rejected.

Doing this cuts us off from our unique talents as well as our ability to transform our lives for the better.

How to identify a disempowering story.

Our disempowering stories stem from our limited perceptions of ourselves. And what we are capable of achieving.

We use disempowering stories to explain 'where we are' and 'how we got here'. Our disempowering stories are an attempt to rationalise why our lives are not working as we would like.

We also use them to justify why our lives can't change.

Our disempowering stories serve us in some way. They are an attempt to keep us safe from the things we are most afraid of.

You can identify a disempowering story by the way it makes you feel.

Pay particular attention when you hear yourself start a sentence with words such as...

"I can't..."
"I won't..."
"I should..."
"I'll never..."
"I'm not..."
"I have to..."

My disempowering stories contained many reasons on why I should give up on my dreams. And settle for my little life instead. Believing these stories kept me stuck in the past and on the path of emotional eating.

On my healing journey I found a willingness to grow beyond my perceived limitations. Whenever I have updated a disempowering story, my life has always improved for the better.

Transforming my disempowering stories has helped me achieve many things. Such as lose weight, heal emotional eating, attend art school, travel the world, become a yoga teacher, write books and start my own business.

Which of your disempowering stories are you ready to transform?

Transform disempowering stories into empowering stories.

Once you have become aware of a disempowering story you can transform it into an empowering one.

Empowering stories begin with the words...

"I can..."
"I am willing..."
"I am able..."
"I am open..."
"Maybe it is possible..."

Here are some examples of 'empowering stories' I used to replace my 'disempowering stories'.

"I can lose weight naturally."

"I am willing to put myself first."

"I am able to make positive changes in my life."

"I am open to trying new foods."

"Maybe it is possible for me Heal Emotional Eating For Good?"

I want you to know that you can choose to tell yourself empowering stories too.

You can embrace new ways of thinking, feeling and acting. You can update your self-talk. You can place your attention upon your dreams rather than your perceived limitations.

The key is to turn down the volume on your disempowering stories and turn the volume up on your empowering ones.

As you tell yourself new empowering stories, look for evidence to confirm your life is changing for the better.

This will help to reduce any resistance you might initially feel. As well as help you to cultivate new levels of self-esteem and confidence.

Stephanie transformed her disempowering stories.

A few months after our *Breakthrough Healing Session*, I had a follow up chat with Stephanie.

She thanked me and told me our session together had given her the boost she had been looking for.

Stephanie shared she had started taking baby steps to bring her body back into balance.

She had cut back on sugar, stopped drinking alcohol and started losing weight.

She had also begun to pay attention to the stories she had been telling herself.

Any time she felt an urge for emotional eating, she would pause and notice her thoughts.

If she caught herself telling a disempowering story, she would remind herself she didn't have to believe it.

Once she had noticed a disempowering story she would write it down in her journal. Then using her imagination she would transform it into an empowering story. One that was more aligned with what she wanted.

She also used affirmations to remind herself that healing is a journey.

She shared she had released her disempowering story about not having support. Instead she was now focused upon assembling her *"Healing Dream Team"*.

She had given herself permission to be open and vulnerable. She was amazed at how the people in her life were responding and loved feeling a new depth within her relationships.

She also shared she had joined a local dance class. And was learning how to express her emotions in healthy ways.

Exercise: Transform your disempowering stories.

Affirmations are a great healing tool to help you transform your old disempowering stories. The following list will help you get started. With time you might also like to create your own affirmations.

Healing affirmations for emotional eating.
I am willing to change.
I am ready to heal.
I release my past with love.
It's safe to let go.
I am willing to trust.
Everything unfolds with divine timing.
I have everything I need.
I love and accept myself.
I approve of myself.
I am worthy and deserving of love.
I treat myself with kindness and compassion.
I eat food that nourishes my body.
My body and mind are working together harmoniously.
It's safe for me to move forward.
I am unique and I am beautiful.
I am whole and complete.
I am good enough.

Live your empowering stories

"If you hear a voice within you saying, 'you are not a painter' then by all means paint and that voice will be silenced."

~ Vincent Van Gogh

After the group leader dropped me off in the middle of the woods, I threw my backpack to the ground and wept...

"You stupid, stupid, stupid girl... You've really outdone yourself this time. You should have known that this camp would turn out to be a total disaster..."

"I mean how could you be so clueless and dim? All the warning signs were there... But you wouldn't listen... And now you are getting exactly what you deserve..."

When this inner voice grew tired of attacking me, it lashed out at my team leader.

"How dare he leave me out here all alone... In the wild... To fend for myself... Doesn't he know that he is putting my life at risk? What kind of person would do that? I knew I should never have trusted him."

All these inner theatrics carried on until the sun started to set.

Sure enough my inner survivalist kicked in. It was late in the day and I had little choice other than to set up camp.

I begrudgingly grabbed the tarp and rope. After a couple of fruitless attempts, I managed to string the black plastic up around some trees. I then lay my sleeping mat and bag underneath it.

I stood back and admired my handy work. I then mused to myself *"Maybe I could make a go of this living in the bush thing?"*

My shelter was sorted. I just prayed it wouldn't rain for the following 48 hours...

My next task was to create a campfire.

I scanned the surrounding woods for rocks to construct my fire pit.

I needed stones big enough to contain the flames yet easy enough for me to carry. I managed to find some scattered close by.

I had to laugh at myself as I fashioned them into a stone circle.

I felt like some kind of cave woman working with the natural elements left out for me by the gods.

I then turned my attention to gathering dry firewood. I picked up fallen branches, sticks, twigs, leaves, bark and logs from the forest floor.

I assembled my raw materials into a stack inside the pit. I tore a piece of paper out of my journal, scrunched it up loosely and pushed it into the pile.

I took a deep breath and struck a match. I then gently edged it towards a corner of the blank page.

The paper burst into a blue white flame. It caught the kindling and turned tangerine. Soon I was basking in glowing embers.

The fire began to roar as nightfall settled in.

The scene was remarkably similar to the vision I had seen in my dream.

Admittedly my oatmeal cookie wasn't quite as exciting as toasting marshmallows. But I enjoyed it nonetheless.

A spontaneous smile erupted over my face as the stars in the night sky twinkled above me. I was feeling tender yet unexpectedly euphoric.

Silent tears of elation streamed down my face as I sat mesmerised by the dancing flames.

Even the owls seemed to cheer me on as they hooted all around me.

I was alone. I was wild. And I was alive.

Enjoying the fruits of courage.

The following morning I awoke to the joyous sound of bird song.

My first breath was filled with the fragrance of wildflowers. Rabbits pranced nearby and butterflies moseyed about all around me.

I had survived the night. I felt jubilant.

After splashing cold water on my face from a nearby stream, I considered my breakfast options.

Carrot or apple? It was a tough call.

I opted for the apple. I sliced it with my pocketknife in an attempt to make it appear more enticing.

It was unlike any apple I had ever tasted before. It was so sweet, juicy and flavoursome. I savoured every morsel. Even my taste buds appeared to be pulsating with an unexpected gratitude.

After breakfast, I took out my journal and started to write about the events from the previous day.

Seeing what I had written down in my journal was very powerful.

I realised if I had listened to my disempowering stories I would have missed out on this incredible high.

Being out in the woods on my own without any distractions was a life changing experience for me.

I could now see how my disempowering stories had kept me living a life stuck inside my comfort zone. I was reminded yet again that it was possible to outgrow the confines of my previous life experience.

It was such a relief to know that I didn't have to believe my thoughts. Finally, I could see them for what they were...

Clouds passing in the sky.

Live your empowering stories.

When you live your empowering stories you will supercharge your journey to *Heal Emotional Eating For Good.*

The key to living your empowering stories is to start from where you are. And then begin taking baby steps in the direction of your dreams.

Celebrate every small victory you experience along your journey. As you do, your courage, confidence and conviction will grow.

With practice you will find yourself effortlessly handling setbacks and obstacles in your life.

Not only will you be dealing with these challenges, they will make you stronger.

People and situations that would have triggered your emotional eating in the past, will no longer affect you.

Even your taste buds will begin to change.

You will notice that real food prepared with love tastes better than anything else in the world. You will also connect with the joy that comes from moving your body in fun and flowing ways.

Telling empowering stories will soon become a habit and an everyday part of your reality.

So too will expressing gratitude for life's many blessings.

You will start to attract all the support and resources you need to be successful. Momentum will follow as you focus upon creating the life you desire.

Your hopes and dreams will begin to manifest. And you will achieve things you never thought possible...

Chapter summary.

To *Heal Emotional Eating For Good* it is important you become the author and creator of your own life.

Healing happens as you build awareness of the stories you tell yourself.

Notice the impact they have upon the way you feel as well as your food choices.

Once you become aware of a disempowering story, you can update it into a story that inspires and empowers.

Transform your stories with healing tools like journaling and affirmations.

Your future possibilities do not have to be dictated by your past.

Instead begin to imagine the exciting new possibilities that await you.

When you live your empowering stories you energise your dreams rather than your fears and doubts.

This will help you to refocus, reprioritise and reorganise your life around what is most important to you.

Your empowering stories provide evidence you have what it takes to heal. And be successful in your life.

Rather than feeling overwhelmed you will feel motivated to make positive change.

Remember that your stories have power.

Use them with awareness to *Heal Emotional Eating For Good* and to create the life you have always dreamed of.

PHASE 3:

Emotional Freedom

Chapter Ten – Living Your Dreams

"The privilege of a lifetime is being who you are."

~ Joseph Campbell

How will I know I have healed emotional eating?

"Maybe the journey isn't so much about becoming anything. Maybe it's about unbecoming everything that isn't you so you can be who you were meant to be in the first place."

~ Unknown

Well done on making it to Phase 3 and the final chapter of this book.

I remember hearing somebody, somewhere tell me that most people don't get past the first chapter of the books they read.

As an author, I have to admit this felt a little disheartening to hear at the time.

As I reflected on this statement, it started to make sense why this might be the case.

We live in a busy world. With so many things competing for our time and attention it's easy to get distracted.

My reflections also made me even more appreciative of the women who take the time to read what I write.

Whether it be an article on my blog or a chapter from one of my books, I am filled with gratitude.

The fact you are still here with me reading this final phase is an extra special blessing.

So I want to acknowledge you for making it this far.

It says a lot about you and your willingness to take the steps necessary to change your life for the better.

I know this determination and persistence will be a great asset to you on your healing journey.

I recently had a lovely conversation with a woman about my work and my first book *Losing Weight is a Healing Journey*.

Whilst chatting, I mentioned I was writing my second book *Heal Emotional Eating For Good*.

"What an interesting title" she said. *"Do you mind if I ask you a personal question?"*

"Sure" I said.

"So how did you know you had healed your emotional eating?"

"Well to be honest, at first, I didn't even know it was possible to heal emotional eating." I replied.

"For years, I was wrapped up in the myths of the dieting model. I used to think I would be able to control my food cravings if I had more discipline or willpower."

"Rather than help me, this approach intensified my struggle with emotional eating."

"Feeling as if I had 'failed at dieting' deepened my sense of shame and inadequacy. Like there must be something wrong with me..."

"I carried on suppressing my feelings with food and soothing my uncomfortable emotions. Sure enough, my body kept giving me signs it wasn't happy either..."

"Of course I didn't listen and carried on struggling with my emotional eating. All this did was throw my body even further out of balance. And then one day, my body signaled it had finally had enough."

"My body breakdown was the most humbling moment of my life. It also became the start of my healing journey..."

"I was sick, tired and 60lbs overweight. I had no idea how I was going to turn my life around. I wasn't even sure if it was possible."

"What I did know was that I had chosen to heal my life."

"Fortunately I met a healing guide..."

"She introduced me to a whole new way of being. She helped me to see that my excess weight and emotional eating weren't the real problem. They were symptoms of it."

"This new awareness sparked something within me. I began to realise my food cravings weren't something I needed to suppress or control."

"Instead they were something to pay attention and listen to. They became a gentle reminder that I had healing work to do."

"I decided to use my emotional eating as an opportunity to look within and discover what was going on in my life."

"I began to see I hadn't been living a life that was true to me."

"I had been so focused upon pleasing other people and trying to fit in with society's expectations. I had been neglecting my own needs and this created all kinds of unnecessary stress and anxiety in my life."

"As I progressed on my journey I discovered many healing tools. I used them to release my past and open to new possibilities."

"Although I felt unsure of myself, I took baby steps and noticed what worked for me and also what didn't. 'Progress not perfection' became a healing mantra I would repeat to myself."

"I soon noticed my life was transforming for the better and my confidence started to build. My excess weight began to fall off and I was feeling happier and healthier than ever before."

"I followed my intuition and discovered how to be true to myself. I also learnt how to express my emotions in healthy and creative ways. Best of all, I finally felt comfortable in my own skin."

"One day it dawned on me I no longer needed food to cope with the stress of my everyday life. It was an incredible inner victory. It was in that moment I realised I had healed emotional eating for good."

"And it felt fantastic..."

10 signs you have healed emotional eating for good.

American author Ursula K. Le Guin in her novel *The Left Hand of Darkness* wrote, *"It is good to have an end to journey toward, but it is the journey that matters in the end."*

Your journey to *Heal Emotional Eating For Good* will be a deeply personal one. It will contain failure and success, ups and downs, as well as many unexpected twists and turns.

Like any good journey, what you discover is more important than the ultimate destination.

Here are 10 useful signposts to look for as you progress along your healing journey.

1. You no longer use food to cope with stress. This is the big one. You no longer use fake food as a coping strategy. You have a selection of healing tools you can call upon when you are experiencing emotional stress, discomfort or pain. You use the healing tools most appropriate for the situation.

2. You have released unnecessary stress in your life. You have taken stock of your life and let go of unnecessary stress. You have released toxic foods, friendships, relationships, habits and beliefs that no longer serve you. You also choose to spend time with people who uplift and inspire you.

3. You have released your clutter. You have removed clutter from your environment. Including your home, workplace, garage, car, storage units and even your handbag. You now surround yourself with things you use and love. You no longer feel the need to fill your life with meaningless stuff. You have also created space for more joy to flow into your life.

4. You have set up your kitchen for success. You have organised your kitchen for success and to make healthy eating effortless. Your kitchen is well stocked with healthy ingredients. You know where everything is and can access the right kitchen equipment easily. You have substituted fake foods in your pantry with healthy alternatives.

5. You treat your body with respect. You love your body and give it the care that it deserves. You have released excess weight and have brought your body back into balance. You nourish your body with real foods, clean water and gentle movement. You also give it the sleep and rest it needs. Your body is the sacred temple for your soul and you are filled with gratitude for everything that it does for you.

6. You have cultivated a peaceful relationship with food. You no longer obsess over food. You eat when you are hungry and stop when you are full. You prefer to eat fresh, healthy food because it tastes better than anything else. You attune to the wisdom of your body and eat foods that are right for you. You know there is no need for struggle. Your food choices are aligned with your health and wellbeing.

7. You express yourself in healthy ways. You no longer use fake food to suppress or repress difficult thoughts and feelings. Instead, you use healing tools to acknowledge and release them. You have transformed self-sabotage patterns into creative life force energy. So that you can manifest your deepest desires.

8. You have released your pain. You have used healing tools to release emotional wounds from your past. You no longer feel the need to cling to old disempowering stories. You learn from all your life experiences and use the lessons to become a better person. By releasing the pain of your past, you create space for the person you are becoming.

9. You have healed your relationship with others. You have made peace with the people that have hurt or upset you in your life. You have forgiven them for any harm they may have caused. You have used your past life experiences to grow wiser. You no longer take things personally. This wisdom helps you to create a life filled with hope, health and happiness.

10. You have healed your relationship with yourself. You have entered into a more honest, loving and empowered relationship with yourself. You have increased your levels of self-awareness. You now have a better understanding of your natural talents as well as your limitations. You no longer seek fulfillment through empty calories. Instead you give yourself permission to listen to your intuition and go after your dreams.

Exercise: Healing self-assessment tool.

Use the following self-assessment tool to gauge your progress as you *Heal Emotional Eating For Good.*

Healing doesn't happen in a straight line. Focus upon 'progress not perfection' and be patient and gentle with yourself.

As you do your healing work, be on the look out for blessings and surprise synchronicities to show up in your life.

And most importantly celebrate every baby step you make along your healing journey.

Check the following statements to see if they feel true for you...

Healing self-assessment tool.	Yes / No
1. I no longer use food to cope with stress.	
2. I have eliminated unnecessary stress in my life.	
3. I have released my clutter.	
4. I have set up my kitchen for success.	
5. I treat my body with love and respect.	
6. I enjoy a peaceful relationship with food.	
7. I express myself in healthy ways.	
8. I have released my pain.	
9. I have healed my relationship with others.	
10. I have healed my relationship with myself.	

Live a life you love

"Let yourself be silently drawn by the strange pull of what you really love. It will not lead you astray."

~ Rumi

When I look back at my emotional eating and weight challenges, I am filled with gratitude.

Yes it was a very difficult period in my life.

And no, I wouldn't have it any other way.

The earlier version of me would have found it hard to believe I would one day feel grateful for my challenges.

Before going on my healing journey, my emotional eating and weight problems seemed insurmountable.

Like a battle I was going to struggle with for the rest of my life.

With the benefit of hindsight, I can now see the challenges I faced were there to help me grow.

Each time I stumbled on the path, it strengthened my resolve to *Heal Emotional Eating For Good.*

It seems strange I had to struggle through that difficult period to transform my life.

Like a caterpillar unknowingly spinning herself into the confines of a silk cocoon. So she could one day emerge as a beautiful butterfly.

The amazing thing was, I did come out on the other side.

Even though there were plenty of moments when this seemed like the most unlikely thing in the world...

And I know it is possible for you too.

My healing journey helped me become aware of the patterns, programs and beliefs keeping me stuck.

The main reason why they had become so painful was because I had outgrown them.

They were like a pair of shoes that no longer fit. The more I tried to squeeze back into them, the more pain they caused.

One thing I learnt on my healing journey is that our pain can be a gift if we allow it to be.

My emotional eating was a knock at the door, inviting me to explore what was possible in my life.

It was the catalyst that helped me to grow beyond the confines of my past and into the person I dreamt of becoming.

In the process I transformed every aspect of my life.

I finally healed my relationship with food. I discovered that the sacred act of eating was never intended to cause me harm.

I found that real foods contained the true nourishment, healing and life force energy I had been searching for.

I learnt how to extend kindness and compassion towards myself.

I befriended my body and embraced my sensitive and creative nature.

I discovered what was important to me. And even connected with personal gifts and talents I didn't know I had.

I surprised myself over and over again.

Our challenges dissolve when we call upon the innate power we have residing within us.

When we connect with our dreams, the whole Universe starts aligning in our favour...

Exercise: Healing visualisation.

Using the power of your imagination is one of the most profound healing tools available.

The following visualisation will help you to connect with new possibilities.

Stay open and playful with this process. It will become easier with practice.

Imagining new possibilities for your life.

I want you to take a moment to imagine what your life will be like once you *Heal Emotional Eating For Good*.

Start by imagining what it would feel like to transform your relationship with food…

Imagine a life where there is no need to go on meaningless diets, count calories or deprive yourself.

What kinds of delicious and wholesome meals will you prepare?

What new foods and recipes will you try?

What would it be like to feel happy and content after you eat?

What would it feel like to have the confidence and courage to speak your truth?

Imagine if you stopped trying to please other people. And instead focused upon being at peace with yourself?

Imagine a life where you didn't have to believe your old stories.

What would become possible if you replaced them with empowering stories instead?

How would you choose to spend your time if you no longer struggled with emotional eating?

Where would you invest your love, energy and attention?

What kind of work would you really love to do?

Maybe you would like to set up a business that inspires hearts and minds around the world? Or start a charity to help others?

Where would you choose to live? Maybe you've always dreamt of living someplace new?

What would your life look like if you committed to having more fun?

Would you play more? Laugh more? Dance more? Sing more?

Would you dedicate more time to expressing your creativity?

Would you establish a regular writing practice? Learn a musical instrument or sign up for a painting class?

Would you love to learn a new language or travel the world?

Perhaps go on a wellness retreat in an exotic location?

Or train as a yoga teacher so you can lead and encourage others?

Maybe you would like to develop deeper connections with your friends and family?

Or find your soul mate?

And what about your spiritual practices?

Would you like to meditate more often? Or perhaps explore and develop your healing gifts?

These things become possible when you realise that emotional eating is not a problem to be solved.

But rather an invitation to live the life of your dreams…

Emotional eating is the doorway to your dreams.

When I started my healing journey I had no idea my emotional eating would end up being the doorway to my dreams.

One of the secrets of healing is to give yourself full permission to do the things you love.

Your emotional eating is a gift to teach you everything you need to be true to yourself.

Allow it to guide you back home towards your intuition and your heart.

Listen to the gentle whispers of your dreams. Allow them to inspire and uplift you to become the best person you can be.

You are here to live an extraordinary life filled with vibrant health and happiness.

Allow your courage to grow bigger than your fears and let your light shine brightly.

I love you.

I believe in you.

I know that you can do this.

I look forward to hearing about your healing journey.

And celebrating your success...

Afterword

"We are told to let our light shine, and if it does, we won't need to tell anybody it does. Lighthouses don't fire cannons to call attention to the shining—they just shine."

~ Dwight L. Moody

There is one last thought I would like to share with you.

When you overcome difficulty and challenge in your life, you have an incredible gift to share with others.

When I was struggling with emotional eating, it was almost impossible for me to imagine I would one day be inspiring other women.

And today paying my blessings forward is my greatest privilege. It is something that creates such purpose and meaning in my life.

This very special possibility also exists inside of you.

Giving back is what completes the virtuous cycle of life.

Once you fill your own cup, allow your beauty and truth to overflow into the world around you.

Go out into the world and share what you have learnt.

Offer the world your happiness.

Allow your bliss to become contagious.

And together we can make this world a better place…

Claim Your FREE Gift

Get Your Healing Meditation Now!

Are you ready to take the next step on your healing journey?

Would you like some extra support to release the stress at the root of emotional eating?

Visit the website below to download your FREE Healing Meditation...

www.HealEmotionalEating.net

As a special bonus for downloading the meditation you will also receive access to Katrina's weekly newsletter.

It is filled with useful tips, tools and transformational ideas for your healing journey.

It also includes the latest information on Katrina's upcoming programs, workshops and retreats.

A Favour to Ask

Dear Reader,

Did you enjoy reading this book?

If so, I would really appreciate your help.

Online book reviews play a vital role in helping new readers decide what book to read next.

The more online reviews a book receives, the greater the chance it has to find new readers.

By leaving your review on **www.Amazon.com**, no matter how short, you will be inspiring other women to start their own healing journeys.

You will also be supporting me to continue my work.

Each book review really does make a big difference.

Thank you so much.

Love Katrina xo